The Therapeuti
in Mental Health

A Values-Based and Person-Centered Approach

The Therapeutic Interview in Mental Health

A Values-Based and Person-Centered Approach

Giovanni Stanghellini
Department of Psychological, Humanistic and Territorial Sciences, University of Chieti-Pescara, Chieti, Italy

Milena Mancini
Department of Psychological, Humanistic and Territorial Sciences, University of Chieti-Pescara, Chieti, Italy

CAMBRIDGE
UNIVERSITY PRESS

CAMBRIDGE
UNIVERSITY PRESS

University Printing House, Cambridge CB2 8BS, United Kingdom

One Liberty Plaza, 20th Floor, New York, NY 10006, USA

477 Williamstown Road, Port Melbourne, VIC 3207, Australia

4843/24, 2nd Floor, Ansari Road, Daryaganj, Delhi – 110002, India

79 Anson Road, #06–04/06, Singapore 079906

Cambridge University Press is part of the University of Cambridge.

It furthers the University's mission by disseminating knowledge in the
pursuit of education, learning and research at the highest international levels
of excellence.

www.cambridge.org
Information on this title: www.cambridge.org/9781107499089
DOI: 10.1017/9781316181973

© Giovanni Stanghellini and Milena Mancini 2017

First published 2017

Printed in the United Kingdom by Clays, St Ives plc

A catalogue record for this publication is available from the British Library

Library of Congress Cataloging-in-Publication data
Names: Stanghellini, Giovanni, author. | Mancini, Milena, author.
Title: The therapeutic interview in mental health : a values-based and
person-centered approach / Giovanni Stanghellini, Milena Mancini.
Description: Cambridge, United Kingdom ; New York, NY : Cambridge
University Press, 2017. | Includes bibliographical references and index.
Identifiers: LCCN 2017014554 | ISBN 9781107499089 (pbk. : alk. paper)
Subjects: | MESH: Interview, Psychological | Mental Disorders–diagnosis |
Patient-Centered Care | Psychopathology–methods
Classification: LCC RC473.D54 | NLM WM 143 | DDC 616.89/075–dc23
LC record available at https://lccn.loc.gov/2017014554

ISBN 978–1–107–49908–9 Paperback

id quoque enim non ab nulla ratione videtur

Contents

Preface

There is widespread recognition of the limitations of symptom-focused clinical interviews. The standard interview discourages real dialogue, frustrates the patient's desire to be recognized, and reiterates asymmetry since it affirms the clinician's values, and ignores those of the patient.

The mainstream approach to clinical interviewing is focused on easy-to-assess operationalizable symptoms. This is a practice obviously based on the clinician's values of objectivity and reliability. This "technical" approach downplays subtle anomalies of the patients' experience, regarding them as unreliable, difficult to assess, and unscientific. The consequence is that much of the complexity of living with mental disorders remains unexplored. Thinness of phenotypes and simplification of clinical constructs are the consequences of this. The actual phenomenal universe of "real" mental disorders – the manifold of phenomena experienced by patients in all of their concrete and distinctive features – is considerably larger than that described in current diagnostic manuals.

In the technical approach, the effectiveness of the diagnostic process relies on two domains: diagnostic criteria and the interview method. Operational diagnostic criteria are instrumental in achieving high reliability in the domain of the diagnostic schema, primarily because of their reduction of criterion variance. Structured interview methods help to improve the reliability of diagnostic assignment by reducing information variance. These two domains are coupled in such a way that structured interviews are designed to explore only those symptoms that are relevant to establish a diagnosis according to the diagnostic criteria themselves. The main goal is discovering whether a patient with a given set of signs/symptoms "meets criteria." Accordingly, interviewing is seen as a technique that should conform to the technical-rational paradigm of the natural sciences in which mental health practice as a branch of bio-medicine is positioned and the clinical encounter is thus conceived in terms of a stimulus–response pattern.

As a consequence, a true dialogue between interviewer and interviewee is discouraged, the interviewer "knows" a priori what is relevant to assess, and the interview is conceived as a heavily asymmetric process in which the patient presents the "pieces" of the puzzle and the clinician's task is to build the "whole picture" of the patient's illness. "Procrustean errors" (stretching and trimming the patient's symptomatology to fit criteria) and "tunnel vision" (avoiding the assessment of phenomena not included in standardized interviews) are implied, shared meanings between interviewer and interviewee are assumed and not investigated, and personal narratives are avoided.

There are several damaging consequences to this. One of these is the uncoupling of diagnostic and therapeutic procedures. Symptom assessment and understanding the life-world of the patient come apart. Symptoms are reduced to indexes for diagnosis. An even more alarming consequence of the symptom-focused attitude is that it merely aims at symptom reduction or control. This applies not only to standard psychiatric interviews, but also to a large category of psychotherapeutic ones, especially those whose ambition it is to be acknowledged as "scientific" and "evidence-based." This approach can be iatrogenic rather than helpful since the patient's symptoms are not just accidental anomalies in her existence to be simply diagnosed and eliminated; rather, they are special phenomena through which the hidden, yet operative (and perplexing, or disturbing) dimension of her existence is made manifest (Stanghellini, 2016a). Symptoms present the opportunity for an encounter between the person and her vulnerability. Symptoms offer the prospect of establishing a new kind of meaningfulness in a person's existence.

The therapeutic interview is much more than assessing operationalized symptoms and eliminating them, or reducing their intensity through some kind of therapeutic technique. Rather, it is *a quest for meaning and reciprocal recognition*. It seeks for meaning, order, and value within and throughout ordinary experience and the patient's everyday life. It is a meeting of forms of life – the patient's and the clinician's – each with its system of relevance and meaning structure, stemming from different and sometimes conflicting values. It is the occasion to initiate a shared project of reciprocal understanding between the vulnerable person and the mental health carer. The word "interview" must be taken seriously. For an interview to be a *therapeutic* one, it needs to be an authentic exchange of views between the patient and the clinician.

In this framework, mental health practice is in touch with values-based practice. Values-based practice is a dialogic exercise, a tool for working with complex and conflicting values and as such it is a direct response to and meets head-on the (values-complex) problems presented by mental disorders. It is essential to acknowledge the patient's (and one's own) values in linking up the sciences of medical care effectively with the unique individuals who (as patients, carers, and others) are at the heart of the clinical encounter.

It is important in developing an in-depth awareness of the patient's values not to conflate them with abnormal beliefs, such as delusions. To confuse idiosyncratic values with abnormal beliefs is not only conceptually wrong and ethically inadmissible, it is also therapeutically ineffective. Values are not symptoms to be "killed." They need modulation, therapeutic accommodation with the requirements of reality, not eradication.

The purpose of this book is to ground the practice of the therapeutic interview on a firm epistemological and ethical basis, that is, on key concepts like "subjectivity," "person," "life-world," "emotions," "values," "meaning," "care," and "understanding." This approach builds on patients' individual experiences, their emotions and values, and on the interplay between these, as key aspects of their self-understanding of their sufferings. Understanding is considered the *conditio sine qua non* for therapy. Emotions and values are keys to understanding a person's experiences and actions within the framework of the life-world he or she inhabits.

In this book, a fundamental importance is given to *emotions* as the core of a person's life-world. Emotions play a central role in situating a person and orienting her receptivity, allowing her to see the things that surround her as disclosing certain (and not other) possibilities, i.e. a given set of potential actions. They provide one's orientation in the life-world. They make one turn one's attention to a particular situation or event, to be absorbed by a more or less defined object, and to move (or move away from) in a given direction. Emotions are functional states which motivate and may produce movements (Rosfort and Stanghellini, 2009; Stanghellini and Rosfort, 2013b). They are kinetic, dynamic forces that drive us in our ongoing interactions with the environment (Plutchik, 1980; Sheets-Johnstone, 1999a, 1999b) and protentional states which project the person into the future providing a felt readiness for action (Gallagher, 2005).

The role that the *values* have in putting the meaning of experiences into order is also emphasized. Values are all that matters to a given person. Based on emotional experience, they are attitudes that regulate meaning-bestowing and the significant actions of the person, being organized into concepts that do not arise from rational activity but rather within the sphere of feeling. Thus, grasping the values of a person is a key to understanding her way of interpreting her experience and representing herself. In general, emotions and values are keys to understanding a given "form of life" or "being in the world," since they contribute to establishing the "pragmatic motive" and the "system of relevance" that determine the meaning structure of the world a person lives in, and which regulate her style of experience and action (Figure 0.1). Understanding a person means understanding the pragmatic motive and the system of relevance that make her behave in a given way.

There is another reason to recognize the patient's values. Conflicts of values are part and parcel of being human. Some of them have no satisfactory solution. This view is the starting point to develop an idea of care based on value-acknowledgment and value-pluralism. People have reasons to live that differ from individual to individual. This statement reflects the ideal of *modus vivendi* (Gray, 2010), whose aim is not looking for consensus about the best values, or sharing common values in order to live together in peace. Rather, it aims to find terms on which different forms of life can coexist. The practice that derives from this supports the patient in the search for value-acknowledgment, that is, insight, understanding, resilience, and development of self-management abilities, rather than merely focusing on symptom assessment and reduction. Also, this practice enhances value-pluralism, that is, an idea of care that aims at a relation of coexistence rather than consensus.

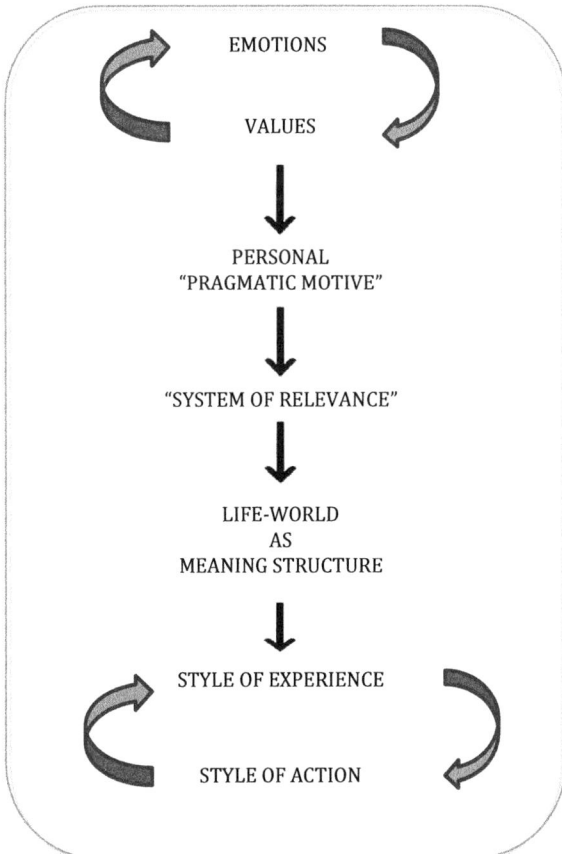

Figure 0.1 Steps to the genesis of the life-world

Most of our current, supposedly humanitarian or dialogic therapeutic practices are based on the ideal of establishing some form of consensus between patients and carers. Yet consensus is a woolly kind of dialogic value. While it looks for agreement and harmony, it implicitly holds that some values are better than others and builds on the metaphysical belief that conflict of values is just a stage on the way to sharing universal values. In this vein, conflicts of values are signs of imperfection, rather a constitutive part of human life. This unrealistic idea promotes pseudo-dialogic practices that downplay the person's subjectivity and surreptitiously endorse one-sided values. Examples of this are social rehabilitation (which endorses prevailing social values), or potentially intolerant techniques to enhance compliance (which endorse the distinction illness/health based on the clinician's values) – both taking for granted that "good" values are on the side of the clinician. Coexistence with mental sufferers and with the values each of them embodies is better practice. This practice is produced in dialogue, which is contact across a distance. It aims to acknowledge, understand, and respect different ways of life, enlighten our ethical conflicts, honor conflicting values – and ultimately negotiate reciprocal recognition (Figure 0.2).

We wrote this book to show how the art of asking questions can be therapeutic. The first part of this book can be seen as the *toolbox* section – it is about the questions to be asked in order to explore and make sense of the life-world each patient lives in. We will provide practical guidelines for performing the therapeutic interview. Its main aim is to link interviewing to understanding, and understanding to therapeutic care.

Since the aim of the therapeutic interview is understanding the life-world the patients live in, the second part contains *cartography* of the patients' life-worlds. The topic of the second part will be the description of the principal prototypes of the psychopathological life-worlds. It contains a map of the answers one may expect while interviewing a person according to the principles illustrated in the first part.

Both are shamefully incomplete, but especially the second part has the most serious limitations. Its intent is to depict the life-worlds of people affected by the most severe forms of mental disorders. As a consequence it does not include several other forms of miscarried existence, especially those which are closer to the psychopathology of everyday life. Also, those forms that are thematically described have simply a prototypical value since we were not able to illustrate the manifold nuances that are proper to each individual existence.

Yet we hope that the reader will learn something from this, namely that interviewing a patient is not merely assessing symptoms and establishing a diagnosis, but a special kind of dialogue between two human beings who share the project of making sense of the sufferings that affect the more vulnerable of them. Not an ordinary kind of dialogue, but a dialogue

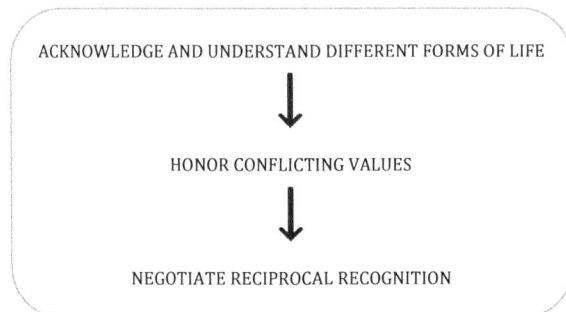

Figure 0.2 Aims of the therapeutic interview

ACKNOWLEDGE AND UNDERSTAND DIFFERENT FORMS OF LIFE

↓

HONOR CONFLICTING VALUES

↓

NEGOTIATE RECIPROCAL RECOGNITION

with a method – a method that involves clear ethical and epistemological principles. The most fundamental of these principles is that a mental pathology is not a mere aggregate of symptoms but a form of existence embedded in a special kind of world as an experiential whole and a concrete universe of perceptions, uses, and values.

1

The Toolbox

Introduction

Interviewing a patient is obviously a crucial step in the overall clinical process. Notwithstanding this truism, a cursory review of the literature reveals that a majority of authors and researchers are more interested in "what" should be assessed than "how" the assessment should be conducted. One reason for this neglect may be that the skill in asking questions and listening to answers is taken for granted as a commonplace habit of everyday life (Lazarsfeld, 1935). Another cause may be the assumption that interviewing is an art that cannot be taught but only acquired (MacKinnon and Michels, 1971). A third, and perhaps more profound, possibility could be that a critical reappraisal of interview principles and skills may become a rather puzzling enterprise requiring us to rethink some of the basic tenets of mental health care as a science.

Studies concerned with the methodological problems of the psychiatric interview mirror a vexed question within the community of mental health professionals (Shea and Mezzich, 1988; Othmer and Othmer, 2002): Is the psychiatric interview a technique designed to objectively and reliably elicit signs and symptoms that allow nosographical diagnosis, or is it a special instance of interpersonal rapport exploring personal problems, including the problems that arise in this rapport and especially those connected to affective involvement?

Attempts to answer this question have cemented a dichotomy between structured and symptom-oriented approaches, on the one hand, and free format and insight-oriented interview styles, on the other (e.g. Shea, 1988). What is lacking most in studies of both approaches is an analysis of the epistemological and ethical problems related to the clinical interview. A lot of work has been done to conceptually clarify psychiatric nosography and classification (e.g. Sadler, Hulgus, and Agich, 1994), but very little effort has been made to bring to the fore the problems that arise in examining and assessing the patient's behaviors, experiences, and expressions. The therapeutic interview is not merely a clinical problem; rather, it may be considered a philosophical problem. By this we mean that there is a need for a philosophically rich approach to the art of interviewing, especially for the task of exploring the patient's subjectivity.

There are many reasons for this. The most basic of them is that the *objectivity* we require from a given discipline depends on the nature of the phenomena under investigation in this discipline (Gabbani and Stanghellini, 2008). A pathology of the psyche may have clear objective causes, i.e. biological bases, but such natural causes do not make of it simply a natural entity. This is not to deny the causal relevance of functional sub-agencies of our brain, but to insist that the assessment and the comprehension of a pathological psychic state requires a kind of analysis that exceeds the range of a naturalistic approach.

Furthermore, a pathology is not simply an anomaly in the statistical sense at a functional or organic level: a strange deviation from normality would not represent in itself a pathology if this caused an experience felt by the person and recognized by others as a condition of well-being and judged as not being problematic in our shared form of life. A pathology of the psyche constitutes an experienced condition and a family of behaviors, emotions, and beliefs, the peculiar significance of which first and foremost emerges within a personal history and a sociocultural context. Such pathology is, therefore, completely on view only because of what has been called the *personal level of analysis*. It is only at this level that the real correlates of a psychopathological condition can be understood in terms of their peculiar feel, meaning, and value for the subjects affected by them (Stanghellini, 2007).

We acknowledge the primacy of subjective experience over objective behavior. There are many reasons for this. First, subjective experiences are more specific phenomena to establish diagnosis. Second, a careful analysis of subjective experience is probably the only means at our disposal to make sense of otherwise odd and incomprehensible behavior. Last but not least, focusing on subjective experience may be more effective in guiding clinical work, including diagnostic procedures and therapeutic (pharmacotherapeutic, and even more so, psychotherapeutic) decision-making.

In endorsing the legacy of phenomenological psychopathology and its emphasis on the analysis of subjectivity by means of the first-person and second-person mode of understanding, we sketch a framework for the therapeutic interview aimed at a wide-ranging, fine-grained assessment of the patient's morbid subjectivity, not constrained by a priori fixed schemata such as specific rating scales or structured question-and-answer procedures. This approach can provide the background for unfolding the phenomena of the life-world inhabited by the patient, including all those details that resist standard semiological classification; and it can uncover the architectural nexus that lends coherence and continuity to them. Phenomenological psychopathology assumes that the manifold phenomena of a given mental disorder have a meaningful coherence. Rather than being a mere aggregate of symptoms, they form a structure, i.e. a meaningful whole. Also, the method of phenomenological psychopathology is a prerequisite for moving beyond pure static description of the life-world towards the illumination of the structures of subjectivity that generate and structure the phenomenal world.

The therapeutic interview may prove helpful in identifying fringe abnormal phenomena that are not covered by standard assessment procedures which are focused on symptoms relevant for nosographic diagnosis rather than on the reconstruction of the complexities of the patients' subjectivity and life-world. It provides the basis for the assessment of real-world, first-personal experiences since this approach is concerned with bringing to light the typical feature(s) of personal experiences in a given individual to establish objective constructs helpful for clinical practice (Stanghellini and Ballerini, 2008).

Also, reflection on the philosophical resources for the therapeutic interview may help to combat the hegemony of de-narratization in the mainstream biomedical model with its emphasis on matters of fact rather than on intelligible relations. Narrative reasoning is the ability to order the significance of our actions, experiences, and beliefs above the level of the sentence, hence above the level of single experiences. Narratives are also the principal means to integrate the alterity of the symptoms into autobiographical memory, providing temporal and goal structure, combining personal experiences into a coherent story related to the self. Obviously, hermeneutics is a necessary complement to pure phenomenology in this context.

Hermeneutics is also important for rethinking the relation between experience and language – a crucial issue for a discipline like mental health care in which language is not simply a means of expression, but the medium in which the interview takes place. The objectifying procedures of natural science, and their concept of objectivity, prove to be misleading when viewed from the angle that all understanding is verbal. The idea of experience-in-itself is an abstraction. From the angle of hermeneutics, all personal experience is given in the linguistic medium, and from the angle of the second-person mode of understanding all that can be understood of another person's experience is a linguistic event – be it the other person's way of talking about his or her experience, or the way I re-enact through empathy that person's experiences in myself, since also my relation with my own "feel" is given in language.

Hermeneutic thinking is also helpful as an antidote to the dehumanization of psychiatric patients. The preliminary step is the unfolding of the phenomenal world the patient lives in, and the reconstruction of its invisible semantic ordering. The next step consists in rescuing the structures of subjectivity which project the world the patient lives in. A further step in the therapeutic interview is the appropriation by the clinician of the patient's life-world: to appropriate the patient's world means acknowledging that it belongs to the clinician's own possibilities as a vulnerable human being. Appropriation is not assimilation, however, since it preserves the tension between extraneousness and familiarity. Finally, the concept of "importance" stretches the meaning of a given mental symptom to its extremes. The way of being in the world of the individual patient transcends the concrete situation of the patient himself and can thus be envisioned as a universal problem since it belongs to human existence as such. The psychopathological condition of the patient unfolds its revelatory power, and acquires a universal meaning that sheds light on the *condició humana*.

In this section of the book we will first review the basic tenets of mainstream interviewing techniques – the so-called technical approach – highlighting their main drawbacks and limitations. Since the interview is, first and foremost, a search for symptoms, we will then spend considerable time analyzing the different ways of conceptualizing symptoms in the bio-medical, psychodynamic, and phenomenological-hermeneutical paradigms.

The next step will be describing the family of tools in use during the interview. We will first illustrate the concept of "life-world" and provide a method to explore it. A psychopathological syndrome is not simply a casual association of (abnormal) phenomena; the manifold (abnormal) phenomena in a syndrome are meaningfully interconnected, that is, they form a structure. This structure is the life-world in which the patient lives. We will focus on two core features of the patient's life-world: their emotions and values. Emotions play a fundamental role in the constitution of the patient's life-world. The patient's values are also of great importance in gaining insight into the patient's way of being in the world as a personal form of life rather than as a mere aggregate of abnormal phenomena.

We will conclude this section of the book with a chapter on the "PHD" method, which brings together phenomenology, hermeneutics, and psycho-dynamics, and a "decalogue" for the therapeutic interview as a quest for meaning.

The Technical Approach to Interviewing

In 1963, an article appeared in the *New York Post* in which the reporter wrote: "a young doctor at Columbia University's New York State Psychiatric Institute has developed a tool that may become the psychiatrist's thermometer and microscope and X-ray machine rolled into one" (Spitzer, 1983: 400). The young doctor was Robert Spitzer and the tool was the structured interview for the assessment of psychiatric symptoms.

Since the early 1970s, mental health professionals endorsing the bio-medical paradigm have increasingly emphasized the need for standardization in psychiatric interviews (Endicott and Spitzer, 1978). The magnitude of the variability between observers in research and clinical settings (Saghir, 1971) was viewed as the main obstacle to the advancement of psychiatry as a scientific discipline. The variability of psychiatric diagnoses had become symbolic of the professionals' self-doubts and of the vulnerability of psychiatry to scientific and public criticism (Kirk and Kutchins, 1992). A consensus emerged among professionals that standardized procedures would eliminate the disarray that characterized the practice of psychiatric diagnosis (Bayer and Spitzer, 1985). Improvement of the validity of the diagnostic schema and the reliability of the diagnostic method became a valued goal in itself (Spitzer, 2001). Since that time, the importance of reliable assessment of psychiatric diagnosis has been taken for granted and become undisputed (Ventura et al., 1998).

The technical approach is rooted in the standard view of science, which praises objectivity and rationality. An illness is the sum of its symptoms; the relationship among numbers is represented by a simple additive effect, regardless of reciprocal interactions. The symptoms are represented by the numbers associated with specific abnormal behaviors. Operations (sums, subtractions, logical operations, e.g. equal to or greater than) conducted on these numbers are supposed to reflect actual changes in clinical reality.

In the technical approach (Figure 1.1), the effectiveness of the diagnostic process relies on two domains: operationalized diagnostic criteria and the interview method. Operational criteria are instrumental in achieving high reliability in the domain of the diagnostic schema, primarily because of their reduction of the variance of diagnostic criteria. Structured interview methods help to improve the reliability of diagnostic assignment by reducing the variance of information achieved via the interview (Spitzer, 1983). These two domains are coupled in such a way that structured interviews are designed to explore only those symptoms that are relevant to establish a diagnosis according to the diagnostic criteria themselves. The interviewer's main goal is discovering whether a patient with a given set of signs and symptoms "meets criteria."

Accordingly, interviewing is seen as a technique that should conform to the technical-rational paradigm of natural sciences, namely laboratory techniques in biological sciences, in which psychiatry as a branch of bio-medicine is positioned. Interviewing is conceived as

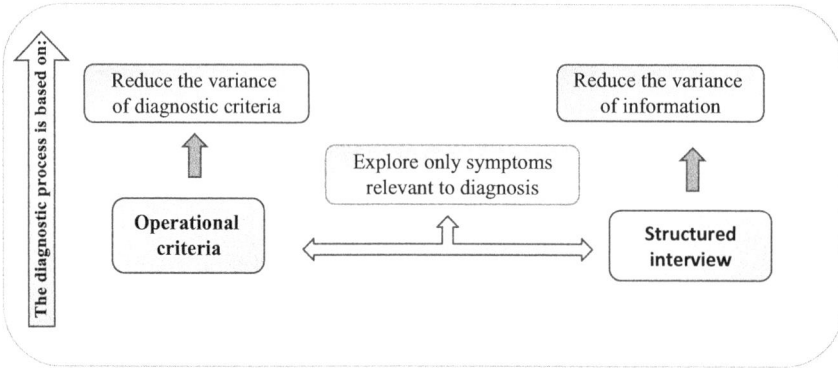

Figure 1.1 The technical approach to interviewing

a stimulus–response pattern of questions formulated in such a way as to reduce information variance (Kirk and Kutchins, 1992) and to elicit only "relevant" answers (Mishler, 1986).

To achieve the aim of reliable nosographical diagnosis, structured interviews are symptom-oriented, rather than insight-oriented. Their aim, or at least their main aim, is not in-depth understanding of personal experiences, but assessing those phenomena that are deemed important as diagnostic indexes. They rely on a descriptive method, and lead to classification of the patient's complaints and dysfunctions according to defined diagnostic categories. The main epistemological tenet is that psychiatric disorders manifest themselves in characteristic sets of signs, symptoms, and behaviors that are in principle accessible to question-and-answer techniques (Othmer and Othmer, 2002).

Early empirical studies comparing structured and unstructured interviews seemed to support the belief that structured interviews are more comprehensive in covering symptomatology and in eliciting factual information and feelings (e.g. Saghir, 1971; Hopkinson, Cox, and Rutter, 1981). After more than 30 years, a large number (if not the majority) of mental health professionals hold the view that structured interviews not only allow better statistical inter-rater agreement, but also, as reported by Ventura et al. (1998), improve non-specialists' assessment in clinical and research settings, permit standardization of formal training programs, and facilitate the development of ultra-rapid diagnosis (Zimmerman, 1993), tele-video psychiatric assessment procedures (Stevens et al., 1999; Yoshino et al., 2001), and computer-assisted or self-administered interviews (Peters and Andrews, 1995).

Ironically, one of the most important unmet needs identified by European residents in psychiatry (Fiorillo et al., 2016) is appropriate training in the use of psychometric tool scales (100 percent of respondents), although these instruments are routinely used in clinical practice especially by early career psychiatrists. It is likely that psychopathological rating scales are often confused with other psychometric tools, which are important for making reliable assessments, but do not explore the patients' perspective, that is, their subjective experiences and personal meanings. Obviously, this deficiency will affect clinical and research work, not to mention the clinicians' epistemological awareness of the limitations of the field of application and of the results obtained using rating scales. For the record, other unmet needs include time dedicated to supervision (90 percent), time dedicated to studying psychopathology (73 percent), and opportunities to discuss patients' psychopathological phenomena in clinical practice (57 percent). The complete list of the results of Fiorillo et al.'s survey of 32 countries is as follows:

- all respondents recognized psychopathology as a core component of training in psychiatry;
- a formal training course in psychopathology is available in 29 out of the 32 surveyed countries but in most countries there is no specified number of hours dedicated to psychopathology;
- teaching is mainly theoretical (96 percent) and discussion of clinical cases is routinely performed in only 24 percent of nations;
- structured training in psychometric tools is available only in ten countries (35 percent), although respondents from 19 countries (73 percent) reported routinely using them in clinical practice, even without formal training;
- trainees consider that the primary aims of studying psychopathology are (a) to assess psychiatric symptoms (47 percent), (b) to understand patients' abnormal experiences (33 percent), and (c) to make nosographical diagnosis (20 percent);
- the most frequently adopted psychopathological approach is the clinical one (65 percent) aimed at nosographical diagnosis, while the phenomenological approach is adopted in 22 percent of countries and the descriptive approach in 18 percent of countries;
- Karl Jaspers, Emil Kraepelin, and Kurt Schneider are listed as the most influential psychopathologists, followed by Eugene Bleuler, Sigmund Freud, and Philippe Pinel;
- at the end of residency, 48 percent of respondents are not satisfied with the training they received in psychopathology; 21 percent believe that psychopathology "is not useful in clinical practice," 25 percent that it "is old-fashioned," and 50 percent that it "is not interesting for psychiatric practice." Six percent of respondents declare having "no time to dedicate to the study of psychopathology";
- the most important unmet needs identified by residents in psychiatry are time dedicated to supervision (90 percent), time dedicated to study psychopathology (73 percent), and opportunities to discuss patients' psychopathological phenomena in clinical practice (57 percent). Other problem areas include lack of supervision, which is available only in 11 of the surveyed countries (35 percent), and lack of training in the use of psychometric tool scales, which in our view should become a compulsory part of residency courses for 100 percent of respondents.

Main Criticisms of the Technical Approach

This approach to the interview, and more generally its advocacy of the assimilation of psychiatry into general medicine as a branch of the natural sciences, has of course raised many criticisms (e.g. Kirk and Kutchins, 1992; Sadler, Hulgus, and Agich, 1994; Richardson, 1996; Stanghellini, 2004; Kendler and Parnas, 2008, 2012).

Procrustean Errors and Tunnel Vision

The technical paradigm conceives interviewing as involving a stimulus–response pattern of questions designed to elicit only relevant answers. It follows a rigid pattern of questions oriented by operationalized criteria for nosographic diagnosis. This may entail so-called "procrustean errors," i.e. "stretching and trimming" the patient's symptomatology to fit criteria (McGuffin and Farmer, 2001), and "tunnel vision" (van Praag et al., 1997), i.e. avoiding the assessment of those phenomena which are not included in standardized interview instruments since they do not reflect operational diagnostic criteria. Both are serious problems; but the second has particularly important theoretical implications, including the perpetuation of systematic inattention to all those features that are not included in mainstream diagnostic schemas, potentially impeding the evolution of psycho-pathological knowledge.

Among these features, the patients' values have a prominent role. But the list of "unattended" features also includes all those subtle phenomena that make up the patient's life-world. The scientific picture of mental disorders seldom presents us with the concrete, real-world picture of the patients' existence. Mainly focusing on full-blown symptoms that are supposed to be relevant for diagnosis, or on subpersonal dysfunctional mechanisms, it downplays more subtle anomalies of patients' experience, regarding them as non-measurable, difficult to assess, and as such somehow unscientific. This is the case of the manifold disturbances of embodiment, lived space, and time (Stanghellini, Ballerini, et al., 2015).

The concept of pheno-phenotype (Stanghellini and Rossi, 2014) may be of help to reinject into current clinical practice (as well as empirical research) important descriptive features that have been marginalized by contemporary overemphasis on behavioral descriptors. This concept aims to describe the phenomenal world of a given patient, i.e. phenomena as they are experienced in the first-person perspective, preserving their peculiar feel, meaning, and value for the patient him- or herself. The utility of the concept of pheno-phenotype (as we will see in great detail in Section 2 of this volume) is to produce a systematic description of subtle and often elusive changes in the person's subjective experience and to reconstruct the ontological framework within which they are generated. This concept is a supportive tool for the phenomenological dissection of psychopathological disorders. The experience of time, space, body, self and others, and their modifications, are the guidelines to this dissection whose aim is to enlarge our awareness of the life-world which people affected by mental disorders live in, understand their behavior and experiences, refine diagnostic criteria, and establish homogeneous categories for neurobiological research. Tunnel vision and procrustean errors reduce validity (Smolik, 1999) as compared with expert clinician ratings.

Obviously, the relevance of some phenomena (and the irrelevance of all the others) is decided a priori – i.e. before the interview with that singular person takes place. The consequence is that a great deal of abnormal phenomena may pass unobserved. The criterion of a priori diagnostic relevance of a given set of symptoms may promote quite perplexing scenarios in the clinical setting. Encouraged by the tenet that inquiring about specific symptoms is a more effective method of conducting a psychiatric interview since it eliminates the vagueness of general questions (Zimmerman, 1993), clinicians may come to endorse a style that transforms the psychiatric interview into a *tele-ocular-dromic* performance: a distancing ("tele"), first-sight ("ocular"), quick ("dromic") scanning of the patient's mental status. But in fact psychiatric patients seem to report a very low number of symptoms in a structured interview that lasts only a few minutes, and the information gathered during this period does not allow accurate diagnosis (Herran et al., 2001).

The Ineffectiveness of Research Interviews for Clinical Practice

The structured interview is a methodology imported into clinical practice from research paradigms, and as such is not responsive to the requirements of clinical settings and the clinician's need. For instance, it deliberately seeks to uncouple assessment procedures (getting information) from therapy, an untenable principle in practicing clinical psychiatry and psychology (Finn and Tonsanger, 1997). Moreover, since it mainly relies on nosographic diagnostic categorization, it may be ineffective in guiding therapeutic (pharmacotherapeutic, and even more psychotherapeutic) decision-making which requires more subtle subgrouping and sometimes trans-nosographical categorization (van Praag et al., 1997).

The Insufficiency of Pure Theoretical Knowledge

To conceive of the interview as a technique entails the presupposition that actual interviewing skills are subservient to cognitive knowledge and the application of diagnostic schemata. This idea has been challenged by several studies: there is a negative correlation between the understanding of interviewing principles and interview performance (Ware, Straussman, and Naftulin, 1971), and a negative correlation between academic (theoretical) knowledge and skill in communicating with patients (practical knowledge) (Pollock, Shanley, and Byrne, 1985). The possibility that cognitive understanding "gets in the way" of clinical performance may indicate that the clinical effectiveness of the interviewing process may entail something more than mere diligence in "learning about" a diagnostic algorithm that guides the interview.

Operational criteria and structured interviews had a positive impact on psychiatry as they contributed to cleanse the earlier profoundly unscientific and irrational attitude towards systematic assessment and diagnosis. Yet, the technical approach to the interview is blind to the essential aspects of the clinical encounter. Subjective and intersubjective features are dismissed even if they have psychopathological meaning. It is this same objectifying intention that compromises the attention needed to notice the aesthetic properties of the clinical encounter and restricts linguistic contexts risking tautology. Atmospheres are examples of such phenomena that should be salvaged to allow in-depth psychopathological assessment (Costa et al., 2014). The clinical encounter is also an aesthetic experience and "tact" as well as technical knowledge is important in sensing atmospheres. Herein resides the need to bring aesthetics into the clinical encounter: one must dodge scientific rationalism in order to preserve phenomenological understanding and achieve an understanding of the meaning of a clinical situation as felt, rather than simply assessing objective signs and symptoms.

The Narrow Dependence on the Standard View of Science

A more global criticism often raised against the technical approach is its narrow dependence on the "received," "standard," or "traditional" view of science (Pidgeon and Henwood, 1996), which values detachment, objectivity, and rationality as guiding principles of Western science. This is the image of true science conveyed to medical students (and psychologists): objects in the natural world enjoy existence independent of human beings (human agency is basically incidental to the objective character of the world out there); scientific knowledge is determined by the actual character of the physical world; science comprises a unitary set of methods and procedures, concerning which there is, by and large, a consensus; and science is an activity which is individualistic and mentalistic (the latter is sometimes expressed as "cognitive") (Woolgar, 1996). This image may well reflect an inaccurate and misleading description of how science actually gets done.

The technical approach to psychiatric interviewing is based on a rationalistic paradigm that is classificatory and explanative in nature as its main aims are to establish diagnosis and look for the causes of a given disordered mental state. As we have seen in the previous section, the conceptual haziness that clouds the idea of "atmosphere" is claimed as good enough reason for its exclusion from scientific paradigms and clinical diagnosis. Yet, the power to appreciate atmospheres may disclose territories of psychopathological understanding that would otherwise remain off-limits. This power is based on the capacity to achieve an understanding of the meaning of a clinical situation as felt, that is, on knowing through feelings, rather than simply assessing objective signs and symptoms. Instead of ruling out the relevance of the clinician's capacity for feeling atmospheres in the clinical encounter as unscientific, we need to devise a method to study scientifically the phenomenon of feeling atmospheres and its reliability in the clinical setting.

The Misunderstanding of Empathy

Another problem with the technical approach is its idiosyncratic understanding of the notion of "empathy." For instance, to Ventura et al. (1998) empathy is the capacity to make emotionally congruent remarks, and Othmer and Othmer (2002) report sentences like "You must feel awful" or "I can see how that shook you up" as instances of empathic responses! Empathy is seen as a special technique to elicit trust in order to achieve rapport and relevant information (Turner and Hersen, 2003), rather than as itself the medium for understanding. In the standard interviewing process, empathy is conceptualized as a way of "putting the patient and yourself at ease" (Othmer and Othmer, 2002) before proceeding to a purely objective assessment. Empathy, that is, is too often conceived as a mere precursor to the genuine article of psychopathological understanding, rather than as one core form that understanding may take.

The phenomenon of empathy is much more complex than that. From a different perspective (Jaspers, 1913/1997; Stanghellini, 2013a; Stanghellini and Rosfort, 2013c), empathy is the basic method of psychopathological assessment that implies the ability to feel oneself into the situation of the other person (Oyebode, 2008).

Empathic understanding can be characterized as a particular kind of intentional experience in which my perception of the other person leads me to grasp (or to feel that I grasp) his or her personal experience. Empathic understanding is the most fundamental method in our attempt to access the disordered mind and involves a continual onslaught on our prejudices (Jaspers, 1913/1997). Nevertheless, empathic understanding can only be a first descriptive step that needs to be combined with a second explanatory attempt to make sense of basic patterns of human life (Jaspers, 1913/1997).

The Avoidance of Subjectivity and the Praise of Objectivity

In the past few decades, an objectifying trend has taken place not only in psychiatry but also in psychology (behaviorism) and the philosophy of mind. This ongoing focus on objectively observable behaviors in contrast to subjective experiences as more reliable indicators of (normal or abnormal) psychic life has been widely criticized (Lieberman, 1989). The celebration of sight as the noblest of the senses was uncritically imported into "psych" sciences from scientistic philosophy as well as from "visually imbued cultural and social practices" (Jay, 1994: 2).

Modern consciousness and sensory reality have gradually developed towards the unrivaled dominance of the sense of vision (Pallasmaa, 1999). We think it is appropriate to challenge the hegemony of vision that predominates today in our culture. We urgently need a diagnosis of the psychosocial pathology of everyday seeing (Levin, 1993; quoted in Pallasmaa, 1999) that has contaminated psychiatry and psychology and a critical understanding of the reasons for this.

Ocularcentrism in psychiatry values a kind of practice that lets the observer avoid direct engagement, helps establish a sharp subject–object distinction, and allows neutrality. The major criticism of this approach is that observable behaviors are mere "shells" whose content (i.e. motivations) is radically underappreciated from a purely "objective," third-person perspective. Behaviors are final common pathways, e.g. anorectic behavior may be motivated by very different mental states like the dread of appearing deformed in one's bodily shape, the delusional fear of being poisoned (sitophobia), the hypochondriacal idea that fat will cause a disease, the value of asceticism, etc. Thus, the category that includes all persons displaying anorectic behavior is highly non-specific and has very low clinical utility, whereas in order to establish homogeneous categories we must take into account the mental states that subtend (abnormal) behaviors.

The Objectification of Subjectivity

Another substantial criticism of the objectifying trend is evident in its avoidance of complex problems entailed by the exploration of subjectivity. It is questionable whether we do, in the ordinary sense, have empirical knowledge of the mental states of others and also of our own mental states. Mental states are subjective, i.e. I have direct access to my own and only to my own inner ("private") experience. But for me to access the complex features (e.g. emotional nuances, motivations, etc.) of my own experiences can be highly problematic. For instance, it may necessitate my taking a third-person perspective on my own mental states and, so to say, to explore myself from without. The objectification of subjectivity may occur in the process of reflection, since reflection implies a third-person approach to oneself. Also, it may occur in the phenomenon of remembering – how does someone remember her past experiences as her own? Does remembering also imply a third-person perspective on oneself? A second shift from first-person to third-person perspective is obviously entailed when someone asks me to explicate my mental states, and this step can be even more problematic. As Zahavi (1999) puts it: Can subjectivity be made accessible for direct theoretical examination, or does such examination necessarily imply an objectivization and consequently a falsification? This is the fundamental issue addressed by phenomenology, namely how to approach consciousness. This shift is nonetheless necessary if we want to assess (e.g. measure) subjective phenomena underlying objective behaviors. The facts that a subjective mental state may be opaque to its owner, and that errors in translation may occur in the process of assessing someone else's mental states, do not seem to represent sufficient arguments for excluding subjectivity from the "objects" of psychology and psychopathology and for confining psychological and psychopathological sciences to the realm of the objectively observable.

Also, mental states are meaningful, and the meaning of a person's action is not visible, as is clear in the case of anorectic behavior. Mental states are subjective, and their complete content often cannot be captured simply by observing the behaviors in which they are expressed at any one time. Avoiding the exploration of human subjectivity is certainly not the best solution to these difficulties. The purpose of the interview (to quote Paul Klee's famous formula) is not simply to render the visible, but *to render visible*.

The Place of Language

The exploration of subjectivity takes place in language. Words are one of the means through which currently opaque meanings are rendered more sensible. Here is raised a further problem: Can words always aptly express a mental state and its proper meaning? For some mental states (especially psychotic and, even more, pre-psychotic ones) are almost ineffable. The "assessment" of a mental state involves two kinds of reductions. The first is performed by the speaker who tries to find the propositional correlate of a given mental state, or the "right words" to communicate it. The other reduction is performed by the listener who must sometimes interpret the speaker's meaning by asking the speaker and himself "what does he mean by that?" This problem, which plagues psychopathological research and clinical practice, becomes even more acute in using standardized assessment, since when interviewees respond to questionnaires, they might have very different understandings of the questions, and this may lead to the inaccurate conclusion that different individuals or groups have similar experiences or beliefs.

An interview is a linguistic event. It is not a behavioral–verbal interchange simply mediated by language. Rather, it happens in language. Language is not a set of formal classes or boxes that we apply to reality (be it inner or outer reality) from without, but rather a medium where I and world meet (Gadamer, 2004). Language is the house we all live in. This has several implications in the interview. First, language is not given as the "reflection" of something or the "mirror" of reality, be it external or internal reality.

Although we do very often use language to represent, this does not mean that language can be understood as a representation of a world whose structure it reflects or mirrors (Rorty, 1981). Rather than reflecting, language instead often "unconceals" (Heidegger, 1927/1962) or "approximates" a given phenomenon. The interviewer approximates the patient's world by means of his own imagination. When he tries to make sense of the patient's otherwise absurd and otherwise meaningless behavior, he must imagine himself as if he were living in a world that is like the patient's own world. This approximation to the patient's life-world is carried out by the interviewer via as-if experiments which are metaphorically expressed: "You say you feel all the others look at you when you are in a public place. If I put myself in your shoes, I feel I'm being *pierced* by the others' gaze," "You say you're always lagging behind your plans. If I put myself in your shoes, I feel exhausted, it's always like *running after* a departing train," etc.

The leading role of metaphors in the process of the therapeutic interview aimed at understanding a given way of being in the world (or a given atmosphere) contrasts with the ordinary use of language in standard technical interviews (Costa et al., 2014). In the attempt to get closer to the personal feel and meaning of an experience, metaphors enable a self-sustaining process of understanding and experiencing of one kind of thing in terms of another, which has been considered by Lakoff and Johnson (2008) as the basis of our everyday conceptual system. Sometimes the experiences expressed by patients are not directly accessible by existing concepts, which means that they can only be indirectly made sense of by a process that is metaphoric in nature. This process brings experience to the reflexive realm, but will perpetually remain unfinished, as metaphors do not *pin down* experiences. Rather, they *enhance experiencing*, amplifying them and enchaining other metaphors. Despite the frenzied concern for reliability that has expanded into the privacy of the clinical encounter declaring the third-person paradigm and its outlined preconceived interviews as the representatives of objectivity, mental symptoms are neither strictly objective nor subjective, and rely on a constant negotiation of meaning that necessarily takes place during the clinical encounter (Stanghellini, 2007). This is due to the fact that the basic process by which meaning is constructed is linguistic in nature. Interview techniques designed according to the third-person paradigm focus the clinician's attention on the search for specific symptoms. It is this same intention that compromises the attention needed to notice more subtle nuances of the clinical encounter and restricts linguistic contexts risking tautology.

A special instance of this problem emerges in a consideration of bodily sensations. What is the relationship between metaphors (i.e. the expressions we use to describe our bodily experiences) and bodily experiences themselves? Do metaphors directly arise from bodily sensations? Or are they similes (imperfectly) reflecting bodily experiences? Or, rather, do they partly constitute bodily experiences? Second, when reality comes into language a kind of interpretation is at work; and the words through which reality comes to be understood also necessitate an interpretation.

The patient's use of language is not simply descriptive of her inner experience, but is rather of a piece with it. The way that she lives in language is of a piece with her inner life, her subjectivity. It constitutes the "personal idiom" (Bollas, 2003) of the patient – her unique set of resonances, affordances, and metaphors which strike her and which both express and construct her interiority.

Language does not always and everywhere constitute a universally agreed descriptive (non-expressive, non-metaphorical) medium of exchange, but rather is dwelled in idiosyncratically by its speakers. It is not possible, therefore, to treat a patient's language use as a straightforward reflection of her inner experience. This implies, in practice, that the coding of each item of an interview always requires an (often laborious) process of interpretation – rather than a pseudo-objective simple "ticking."

The Avoidance of Personal Meanings and Narratives

The technical approach to the interview is dominated by de-narratization, i.e. by the neglect of intelligible relations between persons – the interviewer and the interviewee – and between the person's feelings, ideas, perceptions, sensations, etc. Narratives are the ordinary forms through which we attempt to order the sense and meaning of our actions, experiences, and beliefs. Narrative reasoning is the ability to use structure above the level of the sentence, hence above the level of single experiences. Narratives establish a form of organization in autobiographical memory providing temporal and goal structure, combining personal experiences into a coherent story related to the self. Structured interviews are usually not concerned with personal narratives since their aim is usually the assessment of bits of behavior and expression; they thereby avoid the problem of constructing interpersonally shared meanings (Mishler, 1986).

In suppressing the natural occurrence of conversation and substituting for it the stimulus–response process in structured interviews, crucial epistemological and ethical problems arise:

(1) The stimulus–response process disrupts the specific rhythm of natural conversation. A fragmentation of personal experience occurs. The intimacy of the relationship, based on the quality of the concentration of one individual on another and on the capacity to alter previously stated positions, is affected (Zinberg, 1987).

(2) Shared meanings between interviewer and interviewees are assumed, and not investigated in the process of the interview itself. Serious questions should instead be raised about the validity of the assumption of real mutual understanding. Take the following example: one patient says, "I feel depressed." What exactly does she mean by that? Some patients may use the word "depressed" to describe themselves as feeling sad and downhearted, but others may use it to mean that they feel unable to feel, or to convey their sense of inner void, lack of inner nucleus and/or of identity, or feelings of being anonymous or non-existent. This is especially relevant in multicultural societies since mental disorders are often displayed in idiosyncratic culturally bound phenomena.

(3) Answers to questions often display the features of narratives. But in the stimulus–response paradigm the interviewee's narratives are suppressed in that his responses are limited to "relevant" answers to narrowly specified questions. By doing so, storytelling, i.e. the primary way human beings make sense of their experiences by casting them in a narrative form, is discouraged. Thus, the search for understanding, i.e. meaningfulness and coherence, is discouraged; this process may even be iatrogenic.

(4) The idea of a neutral stimulus is chimerical. Every researcher and clinician knows very well that even in the stimulus–response approach interviewers often depart from standard questions. These departures from prescribed questions are not exceptions, but rather representative of a process that is inherent to interviewing, i.e. the matching of perspectives.

The Overwriting of Personal Meanings and Narratives

The technical approach to interviewing may inappropriately assume a priori systems of meanings that can obscure and overwrite personally structured meanings and narratives (Mishler 1986; Pidgeon and Henwood, 1996). These a priori systems of meanings are diagnostic categories. The nosographical approach based on operational criteria for discrete disorders (as we have seen) may force researchers and clinicians to commit procrustean errors. Diagnostic categories are conceptualized as boxes ("category" originally means "box," "container") in which similar objects should find their place. The pattern of interviewer dominance and respondent acquiescence is emphasized and enhanced. This entails a shift from initial extended self-reports to simple a priori "relevant" yes-or-no answers. The relevance and appropriateness of questions and responses in an interview should instead emerge through the discourse itself, i.e. from the shared attempt to arrive at meanings that both interviewer and interviewee can understand. Otherwise a symptom is reduced to the properties that correspond to one category or box.

There is little space for personal meanings and personal narratives in the technical approach, as well as for meanings and narratives negotiated during the psychiatric interview. Also significant is the fact that each psychopathological experience is accompanied by a personal meaning or value that the patient attributes to it; that is, each patient may take a certain position with respect to his or her abnormal experiences. For instance, the very same raw "depressive" experience of a sense of inner void may be rated by different persons either as the effect of a change in one's body and thus explained as the effect of a somatic disease; or as passively suffered, thus leading to apathetic and disorganized behavior; or it may kindle a "fight" reaction, leading to dysphoric mood and auto/hetero-aggressive comportments. Or it may be accompanied by an "exalted" reaction so that the person will say that this experience revealed to him his true nature as a disembodied automaton. The position-taking (meaning and value attribution) of each patient towards his or her experiences is obviously a relevant clinical feature since it shapes distinct clinical pictures and prognoses (Stanghellini, 1997; Stanghellini, Bolton, and Fulford, 2013). Knowing the patient's interpretation of his or her condition also contributes to the design of his or her individual treatment plan (see Chapter 11).

A relevant example can be taken from the psychopathology of schizophrenia (Stanghellini and Rosfort, 2015). The prototypical patient with schizophrenia is characterized by an abnormal sense of self-presence, perspective, and phenomenality (Parnas et al., 1998; Sass and Parnas, 2003; Parnas, 2005; Parnas and Sass, 2011; Henriksen and Parnas, 2012). If we assume that these are the core features of the vulnerability to schizophrenia (as it is assumed that schizophrenia is a disorder of the minimal self paradigm), why are the clinical forms that schizophrenia takes on in different schizophrenic persons then so different? Why do persons who suffer from self-disorders and undergo these kinds of anomalous self, body, and world-experiences develop either a psychotic (e.g. delusional) form of schizophrenia or a non-psychotic, "negative" or "pauci-symptomatic" (Blankenburg, 1971) type of this illness, or a schizotypal personality disorder, characterized for instance by magical thinking but not by disorganized speech, delusions, and hallucinations? Why do delusions in people with schizophrenia take on so many different themes, and not only ontological ones (Stanghellini and Raballo, 2015) but also, for example, persecutory, hypochondriac, of reference, of agnition (filiation), external influence, and so on? If we subscribe to the "one root/many branches" conceptualization of the manifold of schizophrenia, then we must be able to explain why, arising from the common root of self-disorders, schizophrenic phenotypes take on so many different features.

A plausible answer is that self-disorders, being at the core of the vulnerability to schizophrenia, are narrated by different persons in different ways. The person's background of values and beliefs determine what her feeling of depersonalization and derealization *mean* for her. This personal background is a pre-reflective context of meaning and significance within which and against which persons understand themselves, others, and their world. The assessment of this personal background is essential for understanding the kind of narrative a person affected by schizophrenic vulnerability may construe and develop.

The Categorial versus the Typological Approach

A final set of critiques can be posed from a semantic stance. The standard interview is said to rely on categorization, i.e. the recognition of a special particular (e.g. a symptom) as the member of a class of other particulars that share common properties or criteria. Categorization in this sense can be described as the reconstruction of the "identity" of a certain object via the analytical or algorithmic apprehension of its multiple features in a bottom-up inferential process: "this person shows features 'x,' 'y,' and 'z,' therefore it must be my daughter Virginia." This is the way symptomatological-criteriological diagnosis is supposed to work – but in fact it does not work like this.

As a matter of fact, mental health professionals (as all other humans), in their diagnostic efforts, are instead engaged in a typification process (Rosch, 1975; Schwartz and Wiggins,

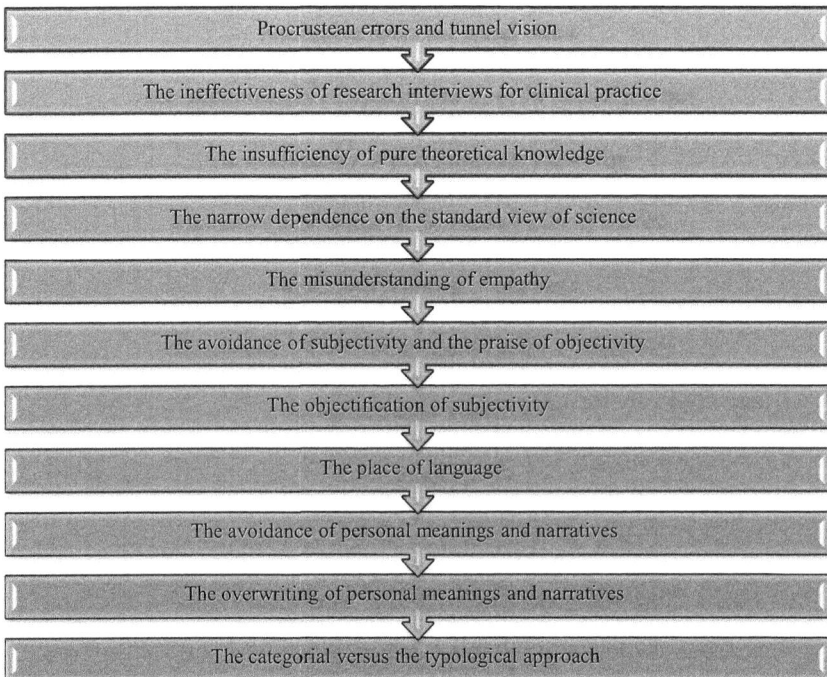

Procrustean errors and tunnel vision

The ineffectiveness of research interviews for clinical practice

The insufficiency of pure theoretical knowledge

The narrow dependence on the standard view of science

The misunderstanding of empathy

The avoidance of subjectivity and the praise of objectivity

The objectification of subjectivity

The place of language

The avoidance of personal meanings and narratives

The overwriting of personal meanings and narratives

The categorial versus the typological approach

Figure 2.1 Main criticisms of the technical approach

1987). Typification implies "seeing as," i.e. perceiving objects, automatically and pre-reflectively, as certain types of objects. The notion of typicality or prototype is crucial here: prototypes are central exemplars. The recognition of an object is founded upon a family resemblance (Wittgenstein, 1953), a network of criss-crossing analogies between the individual members of a category. The typological approach to anomalous experience is concerned with bringing forth the ideally necessary feature(s) of such experience (see e.g. Kraus, 2003). The concept of typification also provides a way to rephrase notions like "intuition" and "holistic approach." The former advocates the primacy of the pre-reflective and implicit over the reflective and explicit cognitive process; the latter emphasizes the importance of the global grasp of a phenomenon as an organizing and meaningful *Gestalt* over a particularistic focus of attention. Figure 2.1 summarizes the main criticisms of the technical approach that we have covered in this chapter.

The Meaning of Symptoms in the Bio-Medical Paradigm

A further set of criticisms of the technical approach stems from its understanding of the concept of "symptom." The technical interview prescribes, first and foremost, a search for symptoms. Handbooks of psychiatry and clinical psychology usually present a list of phenomena that should be assessed and by doing so they establish a system of relevance concerning what should attract the clinician's attention. These relevant phenomena are called "symptoms." Of course, there are different psychopathological paradigms (among which the bio-medical, the psycho-dynamic, the phenomenological, etc.) and each paradigm has its own hierarchy of priorities (what should be the clinician's focus of attention) as well as its own concept of symptom.

One must be aware that the concept of symptom covers a vast array of indexicalities. In biological medicine, a symptom is the epiphenomenon of an underlying pathology. Red, itchy and watery eyes, congestion, runny nose and sneezing, sometimes accompanied by itchy ears and buzzing sound, irritated and sore throat, cough and post-nasal dripping are known to be the manifestation of an inflammation of the respiratory apparatus. But long before we found out what was the cause of these disturbing phenomena (namely rhinovirus infection), we all knew that they were the symptoms of a mild, although distressing and untreatable, disorder called "cold." Within the bio-medical paradigm, a symptom is first of all an *index for diagnosis* used by clinicians to establish that the person who shows that symptom is sick (rather than healthy), and that he or she is affected by a particular illness or disease. The principal utility of any system of medical taxonomy relies on "its capacity to identify specific entities to allow prediction of natural history and response to therapeutic intervention" (Bell, 2010: 1).

The bio-medical understanding of "symptom" is clearly coherent with the technical approach described earlier. Bio-medical research aims to sharpen its tools to establish increasingly more reliable and valid diagnostic criteria. Its real ambition is not simply to establish a diagnosis through the assessment of clinical manifestations (i.e. symptoms), but to discover the causes of these symptoms (aetiology) and the pathway that leads from aetiology to symptoms (pathogenesis). "Ultimately, disease specification should be related to events related to causality rather than simply clinical phenotype" (Bell, 2010: 1). It is assumed that progress in medicine is dependent on defining pathological entities as disease based on aetiology and pathogenetic mechanism – rather than as clinical syndromes based on symptom recognition. So to say, in the bio-medical paradigm the truth about a symptom is its cause. The main, more or less explicit, assumptions in the bio-medical paradigm are the following:

(1) Each symptom must have at least one cause.
(2) This cause lies in some (endogenous or exogenous) noxa affecting the living organism.

(3) The presence of a symptom causes some kind of dysfunction (cause → symptom → dysfunction). Also,

(4) If we want to eliminate a symptom, we should eliminate its cause or interrupt the pathogenetic chain that connects its putative aetiology with the symptom itself.

Thus, the bio-medical paradigm is a knowledge device based on the concept of "causality." In general, causality (in the bio-medical paradigm) goes from aetiology (in our example, the presence of a virus), to symptom(s) (breathing difficulties), to dysfunction (poor physical performance due to blood hypo-oxygenation, thus reduced adaptation of the person to his or her environment). An important, implicit, assumption is also that symptoms are considered accidental, i.e. non-essential to the living organism, whereas the absence of symptoms is considered essential – i.e. normal to living organisms. In other terms, health is considered normal, whereas disease is considered abnormal.

Many of these assumptions – if we apply this paradigm to the field of mental pathology – are at least controversial, or even counterfactual. We will examine some of these controversies later in this chapter. What is of utmost interest here is the fact that in the bio-medical paradigm, symptoms have causes, not meanings. This assumption has been challenged by the psycho-dynamic paradigm. But before we analyze the shift from the bio-medical to the psycho-dynamic concept of "symptom" let's focus for a while on the relationship between symptom and dysfunction with the help of the criticism of the bio-medical paradigm that arises from evolutionary (Darwinian) medicine. Diagnosis, in the bio-medical paradigm, puts emphasis on symptom profiles as symptoms are considered the most proximal indicators of a disorder. From an evolutionary viewpoint, a clinical assessment that focuses exclusively on signs and symptoms limits itself to explaining only partial features of disorders. According to Darwinian psychiatry, clinical assessment should focus primarily on functional capacities and person–environment interactions (Troisi and McGuire, 1998). It is argued that the capacity to achieve biological goals is a better measure of health than the absence of symptoms because it is an indication that the individual possesses those optimal functional capacities that promote biological adaptation. From an evolutionary perspective, not only do symptoms cause dysfunction, but also dysfunction or maladaptation may generate symptoms. When classified from an evolutionary perspective, symptoms can be divided into two broad categories: symptoms as defects in the body's mechanisms and symptoms as useful defenses. For example, seizures, jaundice, coma, and paralysis have apparently no adaptive function and arise from defects in the organism. But

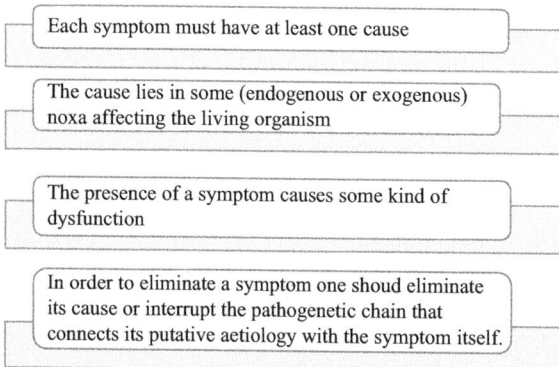

Each symptom must have at least one cause

The cause lies in some (endogenous or exogenous) noxa affecting the living organism

The presence of a symptom causes some kind of dysfunction

In order to eliminate a symptom one shoud eliminate its cause or interrupt the pathogenetic chain that connects its putative aetiology with the symptom itself.

Figure 3.1 "Symptom" in the bio-medical paradigm

many other manifestations of disease are defenses. Vomiting eliminates toxins from the stomach. The low iron levels associated with chronic infection limit the growth of pathogens. Coughing clears foreign matter from the respiratory tract (Troisi, 2011). In the field of mental pathology, it is argued by evolutionary psychiatrists that some depressive symptoms may have adaptive functions serving in the regulation of behavior and psychological processes. For instance, crying elicits comforting behaviors and strengthens social bonds, while pessimism withdraws the individual from current and potential goals. Also, absence of positive emotions discourages approach behavior and risk-taking. More generally we could explain depressive behavior by saying that someone withdraws depressively in order to protect himself socially. Thus, the Darwinian concept of disorder – including mental disorder – encourages clinicians to consider re-prioritizing their selection of diagnostic criteria to ensure that the focus shifts away from mere symptom profiles and more towards comprehensive data collection that includes functional capacities. Figure 3.1 summarizes the conceptualization of "symptom" in the bio-medical paradigm.

The Meaning of Symptoms in the Psycho-Dynamic Paradigm

Early psycho-dynamic conceptualizations of "symptom" address both the cause of a symptom and its meaning. Before Freud, no one asked about the *meaning* of a symptom. Or better: no one posed this question systematically and rigorously. However, since the main aim of early psychoanalytic thinking is to answer the question "What is the origin or cause of this psychical symptom?," it still represents a rather mechanistic view in touch with the bio-medical model. But at the same time early psychoanalysis paved the way for the quest for the meaning of the symptom: "What does that symptom *mean?*" (Stanghellini, 2016a).

Psycho-dynamic thinking develops its genealogy of symptoms around two main pathogenetic devices: trauma and conflict. The psycho-dynamic notion of trauma was first proposed by the French neurologist Jean-Martin Charcot. In 1885 Charcot examined a group of patients who underwent a physical shock and developed a series of motor or sensory symptoms – typically some sort of paralysis or anaesthesia. Charcot's careful medical assessment established that:

(1) The physical shock was very mild and left no traces in the patient's organism, whereas symptoms still persist – these symptoms are (so to say) *sine materia*.

(2) The motor and/or sensory symptoms, their localization, and the way they are correlated with each other, do not correspond to an organic lesion of the nervous system; that is, these symptoms do not correspond to the symptoms one could expect as a consequence of any given lesion of an area of the nervous system. The localization of these symptoms – namely hysterical symptoms – in the patient's body does not reflect the rules of anatomy; rather, these symptoms mirror a kind of imaginary anatomy that imitates true anatomy.

From these observations, Charcot concluded that these symptoms are the outcome not of a physical, but of a psychic, trauma. Hysterical symptoms are not the epiphenomena of a neurological lesion, but rather the manifestation of a psychopathological syndrome. Hysterical symptoms forced Charcot (and later Freud) to see behind the neurological body another kind of body – the "sexual body" (Foucault, 2003). Medicine in general, and psychopathology in particular, from Charcot and Freud onward, must consider the existence of another kind of body, next to the neurological one: this new body is the psychological representation of the body or "representational body" (Leoni, 2008: 18), whose imaginary anatomy does not correspond to the anatomy prescribed by the cortical homunculus discovered by neurology. The representational body, according to Charcot (as explained by Foucault), enters into the mind of a person during a traumatic event and will be inscribed in his cortex "as a kind of permanent injunction" (Foucault, 2003: 274).

Some neurotic symptoms are the outcome of a conflict – typically a conflict between an unconscious drive (e.g. a sexual desire) and a proscription or prohibition by the Ego.

According to classic psycho-dynamic theory (Freud, 1905), this conflict generates anxiety, and anxiety "alerts" the Ego that a defense is necessary. Defenses lead to a compromise between the Ego and the Id. This compromise is the symptom: a symptom is therefore a compromise that at the same time defends the patient from the desire that emerges from the Id, and satisfies this desire in a masked form. Freud (1926: 91) wrote:

> The main characteristics of the formation of symptoms have long since been studied and, I hope, established beyond dispute. A symptom is a sign of, and substitute for, an instinctual satisfaction which has remained in abeyance; it is a consequence of the process of repression. Repression proceeds from the ego when the latter – it may be at the behest of the super-ego – refuses to associate itself with an instinctual cathexis which has been aroused in the id. The ego is able by means of repression to keep the idea which is the vehicle of the reprehensible impulse from becoming conscious. Analysis shows that the idea often persists as an unconscious formation.

It is clear that psycho-dynamically oriented interviews cannot avoid delving into this profound dimension of abnormal behaviors entailing the reconstruction of traumatic events and the unearthing of conflicts. Suppose a young woman develops paraplegia a few days before she is going to get married. Careful medical assessment excludes any sort of neurological deficit. Imagine that through careful interviewing we can ascertain that she suffers from the unconscious desire not to marry her promised husband (or not to get married at all, or to marry another person); and that she cannot manifest this desire, not even to herself. Her symptom, which impedes her walking to the altar, satisfies her desire in a masked form, and at the same time it speaks on behalf of her desire. In this example (if viewed from the psycho-dynamic angle) the symptom has a psychological cause (the conflict) which kindles a pathogenetic cascade (involving a disturbing affect like anxiety alerting defense mechanisms like repression and conversion).

Psycho-dynamic thinking has a number of basic assumptions or postulates. These underlying assumptions are nicely summed up by Brakel (2009):

(1) All psychological events have, at least as one of their causes, a psychological cause, and can thereby be at least in part explained on a psychological basis.

(2) All psychological events can be understood as psychologically meaningful to the person who displays them.

(3) There exists a dynamic unconscious that must be posited because without such a postulate many psychological events are neither psychologically explicable nor psychologically meaningful. In our example, the psychological cause of the young woman's paralysis is the conflict; the meaning of the symptom is her unconscious desire not to get married; and the psycho-dynamic unconscious must be postulated for the symptom to become psychologically explainable and meaningful.

As a consequence of these postulates the psycho-dynamically oriented interview will not merely focus on conscious phenomena like overt symptoms, but will try to elicit unconscious or pre-conscious mental phenomena (e.g. repressed thoughts, representations, fantasies, desires, etc.) by means of free associations (as well as by asking open questions, leaving certain kinds of pauses, not always trying to reduce the patient's anxiety, etc.); also, it will focus on unconscious defense mechanisms (e.g. displacement, idealization, projective identification, etc.), or other subpersonal devices (e.g. attachment styles, self- and other-representations, etc.), as well as on the patient's personal life-history (not merely the medical anamnesis) and interpersonal patterns that will complete the psycho(patho)logical picture. The *Psychodynamic Diagnostic Manual* (PDM Task Force, 2006) clearly states that symptom patterns can only be understood in the context of the personality of the patient and of his mental functioning, since symptom patterns are the explicit expressions of the ways patients face and cope with their life experiences. The reason for this extended assessment beyond mere symptoms or isolated behaviors is essentially practical: treatments that focus only on symptoms are deemed ineffective in producing changes and recovery (Westen, Novotny, and Thompson-Brenner, 2004).

According to the psycho-dynamic paradigm (Figure 4.1), in a symptom, as we saw earlier, an unconscious desire seeks to make itself manifest. What is at stake within a symptom is a repressed desire repugnant to the consciously accepted self-conception and values of the person. This desire, if it is to gain satisfaction, needs to be expressed indirectly. While some symptoms function to express repressed desire (or are a product of defense mechanisms other than repression like projection, projective identification, splitting, etc.), others seem to be "unmentalized" (Fonagy and Target, 1997) fragments of emotions or of self-experience (McDougall, 1996). For instance, one way of understanding a patient who "somatizes" is conceiving of her symptom as a product of anxiety which cannot be understood by the patient and instead is experienced merely bodily. It is as if the meaningful affective component is not simply repressed, but has never really got the chance to develop – because of an inadequate early environment for example.

In contrast to the bio-medical paradigm, and to early psycho-dynamic conceptualizations which were ambivalent about looking for the causes or the meanings of a given symptom, in more recent psycho-dynamic approaches the symptom asks to be heard and deciphered (rather than to be explained and removed).

Lacan's conceptualization of "symptom" is a good example of the turn from searching for the causes of a symptom to searching for its meaning in psychoanalytic thinking. According to Lacan (2005), a symptom (which he spells *sinthome*) is a special kind of speech act through which the unconscious is made manifest. The unconscious itself is structured as a language, and a symptom is a meaningful event. A symptom is a signifier

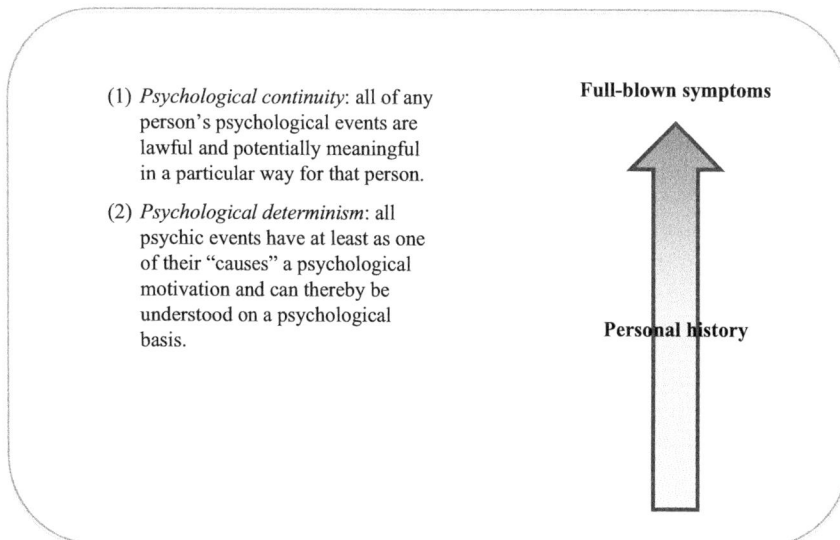

(1) *Psychological continuity*: all of any person's psychological events are lawful and potentially meaningful in a particular way for that person.

(2) *Psychological determinism*: all psychic events have at least as one of their "causes" a psychological motivation and can thereby be understood on a psychological basis.

Full-blown symptoms

Personal history

Figure 4.1 Basic principles of the psycho-dynamic paradigm

that takes the place of a signified that has been repressed. It is a kind of embodied metaphor (Miller, 1998). The Lacanian understanding of "symptom" completely reverses the bio-medical concept. A person's symptom is not accidental to that person; rather it is the manifestation of his or her true identity. Lacan even held that someone's symptom could be the most authentic thing he possesses. A symptom has the same structure of Heidegger's *aletheia* (literally: un-hiddenness). It is the place where truth about oneself manifests while hiding itself. The symptom is not an accident to that person; rather it displays her true essence. As such, it is the contingent opportunity of a possible encounter between the person and the repressed truth of her own desire.

The Symptom as a Text

5

A symptom can also be seen as part of a discourse, to be deployed and analyzed as a *text*.

All human deeds can be produced or reproduced as a text. The text – be it oral or written – is a work of discourse that is produced by an act of exteriorization. One of the main characteristics of a text is that once it is produced it is no longer a private affair, but is in the public domain. It still belongs to the author, but it also stays there independent with respect to the intention of the author (Ricoeur, 1981: 165). The externalization of one's actions, experiences, and beliefs via the production of a text implies their objectification; this objectification entails a distantiation from the person herself and an autonomization of the significance of the text from the intentions of the author. Once produced, the text becomes a matter for public interpretation. Now, the author's meanings and intentions do not exist simply for-himself, but also for-another. This is the point where the therapeutic interview starts: the patient's symptom is no longer a private affair, an "object" that exists solely in the mind of the patient, but a piece of discourse that exists in the context of the interview, that is, in an intermediate space between the person of the patient and the person of the interviewer.

Indeed, there is a parallel between a text and an action because in the same way as a text is detached from its author, an action is detached from its agent and develops consequences of its own (Ricoeur, 1981). Just as every action involves a recoil of unintended implications back upon the actor, every text implies a recoil of unintended meanings back to its author. Like all actions, once produced the text shows the disparity between the author's conscious intentions and unintended consequences.

"All action is a circle wherein our conscious purposes are projected outward, in a deed whose consequences inevitably express something beyond what was intended; the deed therefore recoils back upon the purpose, throwing it into question, exposing the disparity between its intended meaning and its actual outcome" (Berthold-Bond, 1995: 123). This happens because the deed immediately establishes a train of circumstances not directly connected to and contained in the design of the person who committed it. All conscious intentions are "incomplete, unable to anticipate and encompass the full train of consequences, unable through any sheer exertion of will to force the world to become a simple mirror of our purposes" (Berthold-Bond, 1995: 123). The upshot of this is that when we act, via the externalization of our intentions, we may experience a kind of alienation and estrangement from ourselves. We discover alterity within ourselves (Stanghellini, 2016a).

The symptom deployed as a text exposes its author to this very destiny (Ricoeur, 2004; Stanghellini, 2011). A text is the product of an action – a linguistic action. The "mind" cannot see itself until it produces a text objectifying itself in a social act. Because all conscious intentions are incomplete, self-reflection is just an incomplete form of self-knowledge.

A person cannot discern alterity within himself until he has made of himself an external reality by producing a text, and after reflecting upon it. The symptom exposed like a text recoils back upon its author, displaying the discrepancy between the private intended sense and its public tangible result. As a text, in the symptom alterity becomes manifested. The text, as the tangible result of a linguistic act, with its unintended consequences, unfolds the "mind" of the author much more faithfully than a simple act of self-reflection.

This is the effect searched for and produced by the therapeutic interview. Thus, in this framework, the symptom is neither merely an index for diagnosis, nor the outcome of some unconscious mechanism to be repaired. Rather, the symptom is an *opportunity* for the patient to get a new insight about himself. The symptom is the manifestation of a meaning that was not given the opportunity to emerge. It is a meaning (so to say) that cries to be heard. Thus a symptom is a path to self-knowledge and self-acquaintance, the occasion to recognize alterity in oneself. To note, the essential task is not to recover, *behind* the text, the lost intention of the author (as is often the case with the classic psycho-dynamic paradigm). Rather, insofar as the meaning of a text is rendered autonomous with respect to the subjective intention of the author, the essential task is "to unfold, *in front of the text*, the 'world' which it opens up and discloses" (Ricoeur, 1981: 111, emphasis added).

The meaning conveyed by the symptom comes into sight by unfolding the symptom itself as a text in front of me. The meaning of the symptom is not to be looked for inside me, via an act of reflection of the self on itself. Rather, it becomes perspicuous over there, *in front of me*. If I want to grasp the meaning carried by the symptom, I must turn my gaze away from my "mind," and look over there, in front of me.

The unconscious meaning carried by the symptom is laid bare in front of me in the texture of the world, within it, not behind it. As we will see in detail in the next chapter, the symptom is part of the patient's life-world. And the life-world, that is, the world inhabited by the patient, is also a text. The meanings that would remain unnoticed and unconscious to the patient as long as they remain in his "mind" materialize in the world-as-a-text – of which the symptom-as-a-text is a significant component – and become readable and discernible in it. Unconscious meanings come into sight; they materialize in the folds of the world/text the patient has produced.

The symptom, then, is an anomaly, but not an abnormal, aberrant, or insane phenomenon in the strict sense. Rather, it is a salience, a knot in the texture of a person's life-world. It is a place that attracts someone's attention, which catches one's eye, and awakens one's care for oneself in a double sense: since it reflects and reveals alterity in oneself – in it alterity becomes conspicuous; and since from the vantage it offers one can see oneself from another, often radically different and new, perspective.

The unfolding of the life-world as a text makes visible the otherwise invisible texture of the world we inhabit. It makes visible the invisible (unconscious) existential pivot of our experiences, the *punctum caecum* of the person, what the person does not see in herself, and makes it possible for her to see and feel the meanings of her world.

The "unconscious" at issue here – let's call it the *hermeneutic unconscious* – is quite different from the psycho-dynamic unconscious. This is not a *causal* unconscious, rather a *hermeneutic* one. The causal unconscious, as with the psycho-dynamic one, is helpful in making sense of someone's discourse as the involuntary expression of a subpersonal mechanism. The psycho-dynamic unconscious is supposed to *produce* a text, as for instance a slip of the tongue, or dream, or a symptom. Its ambition is building a nomothetic construct bridging an unconscious memory or mechanism and an action that is deployed as a text whose meaning must be traced back to the unconscious itself. This kind of unconscious has the strength of being explicative as well as to allow generalizability.

Although it is a matter of debate whether all psychoanalytic schools share a common ground for a general theory of mind or not, it can be assumed that psychoanalysis, like any scientific theory, has a small number of necessary basic underlying presuppositions. These include psychic continuity, psychic determinism, and the existence of a dynamic, psychologically meaningful unconscious (Brakel, 2009). Psychic continuity presumes some sort of regularity or lawfulness in psychic phenomena and determinism means that the operation of cause and effect is also presumed. To assume psychic continuity then is to take for granted that all of an agent's psychological events – including those that look inconsistent or even incoherent such as symptoms, slips of the tongue, and parapraxes – are regular-lawful in a particular way for that person. Every psychological event can be understood as psychologically meaningful to that individual (Brakel, 2009). This is a basic presupposition that (if Brakel is right) psychoanalysis shares with hermeneutic thinking.

The difference between the psycho-dynamic and the hermeneutic point of view is the following: Whereas, as it seems, for psychoanalysis meaningfulness arises from the discovery of the *causes* of a given act, this is not so for hermeneutic thinking. The third basic assumption of psychoanalysis – the existence of a dynamic unconscious – is posited because without it many psychological events seem neither psychically continuous nor determined. The dynamic unconscious – including unconscious mental processes and unconscious mental contents – is assumed to be necessary in order to explain the causes of psychological events.

The hermeneutic unconscious declines most of the ambitions of the psycho-dynamic theory of the unconscious. Rather than being explicative, more modestly it looks not for past causes but for a present *meaning*; a meaning that becomes visible through the text after the text is produced. It is not supposed that acts and experiences bubble to the surface in a disguised form and that their meaning is hidden in the depth of the unconscious from which they are supposed to arise. Meaningfulness does not arise through the linking of an act or an experience with its unconscious antecedent. Meaningfulness is the becoming manifest of the invisible architecture of a set of acts or experiences. Also, the hermeneutic unconscious "discovers" personal meanings within the text itself, rather than universal symbols behind the text, in the depth of the author's dynamic unconscious.

Chapter

6

The Concept of "Life-World"

As we have seen, symptoms are customarily conceived as state-like indexes for nosographical diagnosis. In the phenomenological-hermeneutical paradigm, symptoms are a special kind of phenomena through which the hidden, yet operative (perplexing and disturbing) dimension of existence is made manifest. They are not accidental to that patient, but rather the manifestation of some implicit quintessential "core" dimension of his subjectivity. The overall change in the fundamental structures of subjectivity transpires through the individual symptoms, but the specificity of the core is only graspable at a more comprehensive structural level. This holistic approach bears little resemblance to the current atomistic operational definitions for several reasons. Abnormal mental conditions are not mere aggregates of symptoms. The actual phenomenal universe of "real" abnormal mental conditions is considerably larger than that described in diagnostic manuals. This suggests a shift of attention from mere symptoms (i.e. state-like indexes for nosographical diagnosis) to a broader range of phenomena that are trait-like features of a given life-world.

The main aim of the therapeutic interview is to obtain a systematic knowledge of the patient's experiences in their peculiar feel, meaning, and value for the persons affected by them. The "object" of the therapeutic interview is the patient's subjectivity, its focus is on the patient's states of mind as they are experienced and narrated by them. It aims to faithfully describe the manifold of phenomena in all of their concrete and distinctive features and to reveal those aspects that other approaches tend to overwrite with their strong theoretical and ontological claims. These concerns are prior to any causal accounts addressing subpersonal mechanisms: theoretical assumptions are minimized and the structures of the patient's experience are prioritized.

This issue can be developed adopting the concept of "life-world." This concept is a supportive tool for producing a systematic description of subtle and often undescribed changes in the patient's subjective experience and to reconstruct the ontological framework within which they are generated.

The life-world is the original domain, the obvious and unquestioned foundation both of all types of everyday acting and thinking and of all scientific theorizing and philosophizing. In its concrete manifestations it exists as the "realm of immediate evidence." The concept of life-world was introduced by Edmund Husserl in his *The Crisis of European Sciences and Transcendental Phenomenology* (1936/1970: 108):

> In whatever way we may be conscious of the world as universal horizon, as coherent universe of existing objects, we, each "I-the-man" and all of us together, belong to the world as living with one another in the world; and the world is our world, valid for our consciousness as existing precisely through this "living together." We, as living in wakeful world-consciousness, are constantly active on the basis of our passive having of the world . . . Obviously this is true

not only for me, the individual ego; rather we, in living together, have the world pre-given in this together, belong, the world as world for all, pre-given with this ontic meaning ... The we-subjectivity ... [is] constantly functioning.

The life-world is a grand theater of objects variously arranged in space and time relative to perceiving subjects. It is already-always there, and is the "ground" for all shared human experience. Husserl's formulation of the life-world was influenced by Wilhelm Dilthey's "life-nexus" (*Lebenszusammenhang*) and Martin Heidegger's Being-in-the-world (*In-der-Welt-Sein*). The concept was further developed by students of Husserl such as Maurice Merleau-Ponty, Jan Patočka, and Alfred Schutz. The life-world can be thought of as the horizon of all our experiences, in the sense that it is that background on which all things appear as themselves and meaningful. The life-world cannot, however, be understood in a purely static manner. It isn't an unchangeable background, but rather a dynamic horizon in which we *live*, and which "lives with us" in the sense that nothing can appear in our life-world except as *lived*.

The most relevant variant of life-world phenomenology was developed by Alfred Schutz (Schutz and Luckmann, 1973: 3): "The reality which seems self-evident to men remaining within the natural attitude ... is the everyday life-world. The region of reality in which man can engage himself and which can change while he operates in it by means of his animate organism. The object and events which are already found in this realm limit his free possibility of action. Only within this realm can one be understood by his fellow-men, and only in it can he work together with them."

A life-world is the province of reality inhabited by a given person, having its own meaning structure and a "style" of subjective experience and action determined by a "pragmatic motive."

Although the majority of people are situated within a shared life-world, there are several other frameworks of experience – for example, fantasy worlds, dream worlds, and psycho-pathological worlds. Abnormal mental phenomena are the expression of a more or less pronounced modification of the ontological framework within which experience is generated. The overall change in the ontological framework of experience transpires through the single symptoms, but the specificity of the core is only graspable at a more comprehensive structural level. The experience of time, space, body, self and others, and their modifications, are the principal indexes of the patient's basic structures of subjectivity within which each single experience is situated (Figure 6.1).

Lived Time

Lived time is not the time of the clock (also named "objective" or "cosmic" time). Lived time is "to live time" (Kupke, 2005). It is the way one feels that time is streaming, i.e. the way we experience time (in a subjective way) rather than the way we observe it on the clock (in an objective way). There can be a deep contrast between the objective order of time and the way we personally experience the duration, flow, and speed of time. Every experience receives its specific significance and value from its temporal profile. Personal time is not homogeneous across the life span or in different states. For instance, youth, *élan*, and health diminish distances for our anticipation. Old age, fatigue, and weakness expand them. Moreover, there is a continuous flow of time in our perception. We live and experience in a state of becoming. Under normal conditions, we let the past be past: we turn to new problems before the old ones have found a "perfect" solution. Our views of the past and of

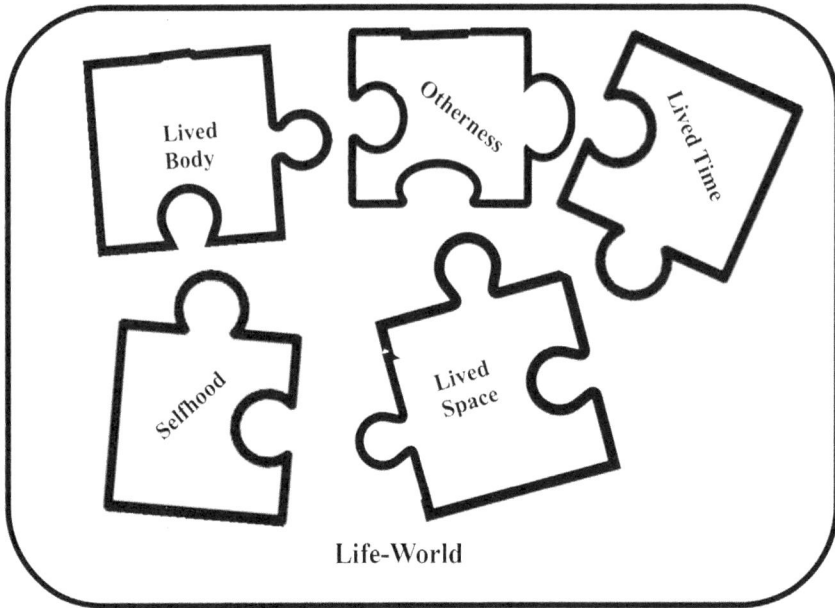

Figure 6.1 Dimensions of the life-world

the future vary with the changes in our state of becoming. Looking backwards on a good day we see the past as a territory which we left behind as a solid ground which supports us; on a bad day we experience the past as a burden which crushes us (Straus, 1947).

Temporality constitutes the bedrock of any experience. It comprises both awareness of external objects and their temporal characters (outer time consciousness) and awareness of one's own stream of consciousness itself (inner time consciousness). The integrity of time consciousness is the condition of possibility of the identity through time of an object of perception as well as of the person who perceives it. Our experience of the permanence in time of a given object whose aspects cannot exist simultaneously but only appear across time (e.g. a melody, or a tridimensional object seen from different perspectives) would be impossible if our consciousness were only aware of what is given in a punctual "now." We can perceive an object as a unitary and identical object because our consciousness is not caught in the "now," but the now-moment has a "width" that extends towards the recollection of the past and the expectation of the future.

Time consciousness has a threefold intentional structure: primal impressions are articulated with the retention of the just-elapsed and the protention or anticipation of the just-about-to-occur. Retention is directed towards the just-elapsed. It allows us to remain aware of what has just sunk into the past. Protention is directed towards the about-to-occur. Unlike retention, which is determinate in content, protention is not filled with a specific content but opens a "cone" of possibilities. It involves a sense of anticipation of what is likely to occur.

Retention and protention should be distinguished from recollection and expectation. These are thematic and, to a certain extent, subject to our will. Recollection and expectation are active doings that we can initiate ourselves, whereas retention and protention are passive processes that take place without our active contribution.

The feel we have of ourselves as unitary subjects of experience permanent through time is due to the integrity of time consciousness. If we have the feel or pre-reflexive awareness of our mental life as a streaming self-awareness this is a consequence of the continuity of inner time consciousness as the innermost structure of our acts of perception. Thanks to the unified, automatic, and pre-reflexive operation of primal impression, protention, and retention underlying our experience of the present our consciousness is internally related to itself and self-affecting (Zahavi, 2003; Thompson, 2007).

Lived time is lived though not necessarily consciously lived (Straus, 1947; Scheler, 1973; Tatossian, 1975). On the first level we find *conscious* time experience. We refer to this feature of temporality with the term "phenomenal" time. Here we find the abnormalities of time experience. The second level is pre-thematic, in the sense that we are not directed to it and it remains in the background of our phenomenal experience. We refer to it as "pre-phenomenal" time (Northoff and Stanghellini, 2016). It "functions" implicitly and automatically (Fuchs, 2013a). It is prior to any active engagement and is involuntary since it does not involve "higher" voluntary level. The pre-phenomenal level is non-experienced but accessible to cognitive reflection.

The pre-phenomenal temporal mode requires two "moments" that can be designated *synthesis* and *conation*. These two moments of temporality are closely intertwined and may only be distinguished conceptually. Together, these moments form the intentional arc of attention, perception, and action that bridges succeeding moments of consciousness by an intentional and affective directedness. At the same time, they are the prerequisites for a basic sense of a coherent self (Fuchs, 2013a, 2013b).

Synthesis produces associative connections bridging succeeding moments of consciousness, namely past, present, and future. The basic temporal unit is not a "knife-edge" present, but a "duration-block." It is a "constitutive flux" that has a dynamic structure that comprises the primal presentation of the now-phase articulated with the retention of the just-elapsed and the protention or anticipation of the just-about-to-occur. The temporal flow of consciousness retains and protends itself and is in this way self-unifying (Thompson, 2007; Northoff, 2014). The "now" does not appear under ordinary circumstances as an isolated, punctual, and unconnected point of experience. Rather, the present moment is like an arrow that has a "whence–wither" dimension. Metaphorically, it has a "width" that stretches towards the just-elapsed and towards the just-about-to-occur. The concept of "synthesis" (Husserl, 1991; Northoff and Stanghellini, 2016) describes the construction of exactly this width with its (virtual) stretches and extensions in our experience of time.

The integrity of synthesis is the condition of possibility of the *permanence* through time of a given object (e.g. the tree that I have *just* perceived is the same as the tree that I am perceiving *now*). It also allows us to properly perceive an "object" that is *extended* in time (e.g. a sentence instead of a disarticulated and thus meaningless succession of phonemes). Last but not least, it allows us to perceive an object as three-dimensional in space through the integration of *perspectives* on the object (e.g. a bricks-and-mortar house instead of a movie scenario).

Our experience of the permanence in time of a given object whose aspects cannot exist simultaneously but only appear across time (a sentence, or a melody) would be impossible if our consciousness were only aware of what is given in a punctual "now." We can perceive an object (a tree, or a chair) as a unitary and identical object because our consciousness is not caught in the "now," but the now-moment has a "width" that extends towards the recollection of past and the expectation of the future. We can perceive something as a concrete, spatially three-dimensional object (a house, or a person), not merely as a "stage trapping," a mere scenario, or a representation of a real thing.

Conscious experience at any moment stretches from the here-and-now backwards to the past and towards the future. This function provides consciousness of the temporal horizon of the present object. No succession or duration, no temporal flux or spatiotemporal perspective, no perception of anything with temporal extension, no experience of three-dimensional objects, no coherence of experience in general, is possible without the temporal synthesis of primal presentational, retentional, and protentional intentions (Husserl, 1991). Had our perception been restricted to what happens right now, we would merely experience isolated, unrelated, punctual conscious states (Zahavi, 2005).

Also the feeling we have of ourselves as unitary subjects of experience remaining permanent through time is due to the integrity of synthesis. When we experience our mental life as a streaming self-awareness this is a consequence of "transcendental temporality," a synthesis which produces associative connections bridging succeeding moments of consciousness, namely past, present, and future and which constitutes the innermost structure of our acts of perception. Thanks to the unified, pre-reflexive (that is, implicit and tacit), operation of primal impression, protention, and retention underlying our experience of the present our consciousness is internally related to itself and self-affecting. Consciousness of worldly objects and self-consciousness and temporality are equiprimordial and co-determined, and phenomenologically co-given in the constitutive flux of consciousness.

"Conation" (from Latin *conatus* = effort, drive) is the basic "energetic momentum" (Fuchs, 2013a) of mental life which can be expressed by concepts such as striving, urge, or *élan*. This concept was originally used in Stoic philosophy and later by Hobbes and Spinoza in particular to denote the living being's striving for self-preservation (*conatus sese conservandi*), in close connection with affective–volitional life. It is given as an experience of *I-can* (Scheler, 1973) that contributes to self- and world-awareness with the sense of aliveness and spontaneity which may be regarded as the essence of subjective life. It also orientates one's awareness in the direction of the future. It is connected with the experience of the person as being driven towards the world in terms of capability and potentiality. The conative momentum is not only an individual, solipsistic force; it is always embedded into one's social relationships to others. We move forward into a promising future because we feel contemporal with caring others who structure the world as an inviting place (Fuchs, 2013a, 2013b). The importance of the conative momentum for the experience of temporality and the self (Kraus, 1996; Svenaeus, 2007) is demonstrated when changes occur in basic motivational states. Examples of this are the acceleration that takes place in manic states or the retardation that occurs in major depression, the standstill of becoming that lets the present and the future be invaded by the past that predominates in depressive states. Both affect the patient's sense of lived time.

Lived Space

Lived space is the way people live space, that is, the totality of the space that a person pre-reflectively "lives" and "experiences." This space is based on the relationship of the person to her world and is embodied in her corporeality. It is the lived experience of space and denotes the world as it is experienced by human beings in the practice of their everyday life. Jaspers mentioned space (and time) as a primary and omnipresent element in the sense world of human beings. Merleau-Ponty (1945/1962) distinguished a physical space construed by perception, a geometrical space conceptually comprehended, and, finally, a lived space. Lived space is distinct from objective or geometrical conceptions of space and it instead refers to egocentric space experienced from a body-centered frame of reference.

As with the experience of time, the experience of space is dependent on the emotions. The way a person is placed in space is nicely encapsulated in the concept of *Befindlichkeit* (Heidegger, 1927/1962) which addresses the way a person is situated according to her emotional tonality. This sets the experience of space in close connection with the possibilities and needs for movement, action, and manipulation, as well as with the appearance and meanings of things in the world.

Lived space has two main experiential dimensions. These include the spatiality of position, i.e. the immediate space of perception and action surrounding the person's body, as well as the spatiality of situation, i.e. the situation of the body confronted with its tasks. In this perspective, lived space is closely intertwined with one's needs and possibilities for action. For instance, things in the world may appear close and ready to be grasped and put to use, or distant, unreachable, and out of touch. Also, they may appear salient, significant, and attractive, or meaningless and irrelevant "objects" simply there in an outer space which appears homogeneous and without any relation with my lived body (see below).

Callieri (2001) writes about the "habitability" (in-dwelling) of space, that is, the space I can inhabit and in which I deploy my own activities. Intuitively, it may seem that the possibility for action is dependent on the experience of space. Affordable actions are those that are allowed by my perception of space and of the things distributed in it. For instance, if I experience things in space as proximate I feel that I can act upon them. Yet the experience of space is also dependent on the possibilities of actions rather than only vice versa (Sheets-Johnstone, 1999b). In this perspective, lived space can be actively structured and organized by the person's possibilities and drives for movement and manipulation.

Under normal conditions, lived space is "not homogeneous, but centered on the person and his body, characterised by qualities such as vicinity or distance, wideness or narrowness, connection or separation, attainability or unattainability" (Fuchs 2007: 426). Each person has a "personal niche" (Willi, 1999), that is, her "working space" in the environment which includes the totality of the relationships with animate and inanimate objects actually present in her surroundings. The person is embedded in a portion of the field as a working space and creates objects for interactive effectiveness (Willi, 1999: 26). In brief, the personal niche is seen as a portion of the psychological environment with which the person is intimately connected and "at home" in: "Niches contain the objects of real and current interactions, against which individuals assess their own reality and receive responses to their effectiveness ... [it] changes continually over time. Individuals are constantly choosing, shaping, and creating for themselves the niches, which in turn form the guidelines for further development over time" (Willi, 1999: 26, 33).

Lived Body

It was Edmund Husserl who first introduced the concept of "lived body." The term "lived body" derives from the German word *Leib*. In German, the term *Leib* is employed when one is referring to living bodies while the term *Körper* is used to designate inanimate or dead bodies such as a rock or a human corpse. Husserl's use of the expression "lived body" was aimed at distinguishing the body that is lived by us from physical bodies. *Leib* is the lived body, the body experienced from within, my own direct experience of my body in the first-person perspective, myself as a spatiotemporal embodied agent in the world. *Körper* is the body thematically investigated from without, as for example by natural sciences such as anatomy and physiology, a third-person perspective. The lived body is strictly related to the concept of lived space, and it is another important aspect for the analysis of the life-world.

Bodily experience, indeed, is the implicit background of our day-to-day experiences against which we develop a coherent sense of self as a unified, bounded entity, naturally immersed in a social world of meaningful others. The lived body is the center of three main dimensions of experience (Stanghellini, 2009): (a) the experience of myself, and especially of the most primitive form of self-awareness; (b) object-experience and meaning-bestowing; (c) the experience of other people, i.e. intersubjectivity.

Self-Awareness

I experience myself as the perspectival origin of my experiences (i.e. perceptions or emotions), actions, and thoughts. This primordial access to myself, or primitive form of egocentricity, must be distinguished from any explicit and thematic form of I-awareness, since it is tacit and implicit, although experientially present. This primitive experience of myself does not arise in reflection, i.e. from a split between an experienced and an experiencing self, but is a pre-reflexive phenomenon. It is also immediate, since it is not inferentially and criterially given. This form of primitive self-awareness is not a conceptual or linguistic representation of oneself, but a primordial contact with oneself or self-affection in which who feels and who is felt are just one thing. Last but not least, it must be also distinguished from a kind of object-awareness, since it does not arise from an objectifying or observational perception of oneself.

The French phenomenologist Michel Henry (1973) uses the term "ipseity" to express this basic or minimal form of self-awareness. Ipseity is the implicit, pre-reflexive, immediate, non-conceptual, non-objectifying, and non-observational sense of existing as a subject of awareness. It is prior to, and a condition of, all other experience.

Two basic and closely related aspects of minimal self-awareness are self-ownership and self-agency. Self-ownership is the pre-reflexive sense that I am the one who is undergoing an experience. Self-agency is the pre-reflexive sense that I am the one who is initiating an action. The immediate awareness of the subjectivity of my experience or action involves that these are in some sense owned and generated by myself. These are the basic components of the experienced differentiation between self and non-self, my self and the object I perceive, and my representation of that object and the object itself. This basic form of self-experience is rooted in one's bodily experience and its situatedness amongst worldly objects and other people. Ipseity is indiscernible from "inhabiting" one's own world, i.e. being engaged and feeling attuned to one's own environment. It is the lived body that provides this engagement and attunement. Being conscious is dwelling in (être-à) the world through one's own lived body (Merleau-Ponty, 1945/1962).

There is good empirical evidence in developmental psychology that newborn infants are already equipped with this minimal form of self-awareness that is embodied and attuned to the world; children, long before they have developed a conceptual image of themselves, have a proprioceptive and ecological sense of their bodily self (Rochat, 2001).

Object-Awareness and Meaning-Bestowing

The power of organizing experience is grounded in motility and perception. A modification in one's lived body implies a modification in the perception of the external world. To Husserl (1912–1915), the shape of material things, just as they stand in front of me in an intuitive way, depends on my configuration, on the configuration of myself as an experiencing embodied subject. By means of the integrity of *kinaesthesia* – the sense of the position and movement of voluntary muscles – my own body is the constant reference of my orientation in the perceptive field. The perceived object gives itself through the integration of a series of prospective appearances.

The lived body is not only the perspectival origin of my perceptions and the locus of their integration, it is the means by which I own the world, inasmuch as it structures and organizes the chances of participating in the field of experience.

The lived body perceives worldly objects as parts of a situation in which it is engaged, of a project to which it is committed, so that its actions are responses to situations rather than reactions to stimuli. The body seeks understanding from the things with which it interacts; the lived body is silently at work whatever I do. I understand my environment as I inhabit it, and the meaningful organization of the field of experience is possible because the active and receptive potentials of my own body are constantly projected into it (Sheets-Johnstone, 1999b). Knowledge is enacted (Varela, Thompson, and Rosch, 1991) or action-specific, and perception is always tangled up with specific possibilities of action (Clark, 1997). Perception is constantly geared up to tracing possibilities for action; these possibilities for action are what we called "meaning," since the meaning of an object is how we put it to use. The basic kind of knowledge I have of objects I encounter in the world is not a kind of mere theoretical cognition, but rather a kind of concern which manipulates things and "puts them to use" (Heidegger, 1927/1962). Objects appear to my embodied self as something "in-order-to," as "equipment," "ready to hand," for manipulating reality and so for cutting, sewing, writing, etc. I literally grasp the meaning of one thing, since this meaning is exactly the specific "manipulability" (*Handlichkeit*) of one thing.

Intersubjectivity

The lived body is also at the center of the problem of intersubjectivity, setting the stage for the understanding of intersubjectivity as intercorporeality, i.e. the immediate, pre-reflexive perceptual linkage between my own and the other's body through which I recognize another being as an alter ego and make sense of his actions. From the angle of intercorporeality, intersubjectivity is a communion of flesh and not a relationship between separate persons. Intercorporeality means the transfer of the corporeal schema, the primary bond of perception by which I recognize others as being similar to myself. This phenomenon is the phenomenal basis of syncretic sociability, i.e. of pathic identification with the other; in a word, of intersubjectivity (Dillon, 1997). Intercorporeality is never fully evident, but it is the bearing support of all interaction connected with behavior, already active and present ahead of any explicit communication. The perceptive bond between myself and another person is based on my ability to identify with the other person's body by means of a primary perceptive tie. Developmental psychologists support the hypothesis that proprioception is involved in understanding other persons through body-to-body attunement (Stern, 1985/2000).

Neuroscientific evidence from neuroimaging also seems to corroborate this view: mirror neurons are a set of visuo-motor neurons in the pre-motor cortex of primates that are supposed to be the neurophysiological substratum for intersubjectivity as intercorporeality. Mirror neurons fire both when a given action is performed by the self and when, performed by another individual, it is simply observed, and as such they are involved in action understanding: meaning is assigned to an observed action by matching it on the same neuronal circuits that may generate it (Gallese and Goldman, 1998; Arbib, 2007).

Selfhood

In everyday experience, we use the word "Self" to define the singularity we each feel ourselves to be, the site from which we perceive the world, and from which we act. We all have a sense of our own self. We often view our self as an enduring structure in which our basic characteristics (ideas, affects, mental processes, etc.) are stored; or at least as a rather stable representation of our own personal identity. The phenomenal self is the self immediately given in subjective experience. My phenomenal self is my present experience of my own body and of the mental events occurring in this moment (thoughts, emotions, feelings), including perceptions of the outer world, memory of the past, and my projections into the future.

The notion of "Self" comprises at least two different dimensions: the pre-reflexive Self and the reflexive Self.

By "pre-reflexive Self" we mean the most primitive form of self-consciousness, acquaintance with an experience (drinking a cup of tea while reading a book, hearing the footsteps of my daughter who is coming back from holiday, feeling excited at what she tells me about her trip) in its first-personal mode of presentation. This primitive experience of oneself is rooted in the lived body. It does not arise in reflection but is pre-reflexive, not inferentiallly or criterially given. It is not a conceptual or linguistic representation of oneself, but a primordial contact with oneself.

Next to this pre-reflexive and non-conceptual dimension of self-consciousness there is an experience of one's own self that implies the possession of a concept of oneself. This is the Self as narrative identity – the Self that tells stories about itself that exists in those stories and conceives its identity in terms of those stories (Phillips, 2003). We will discuss this dimension of the Self in more detail in Chapter 8 and develop here the main dimensions of the pre-reflexive Self.

Traditionally (Jaspers, 1913/1997) self-consciousness is distinguished from object-consciousness (the consciousness we have of external objects, like this book or the easy chair I'm sitting on). Pre-reflexive self-consciousness is defined according to four formal characteristics:

(i) self-consciousness in contrast to the external world and to others;

(ii) sense of activity;

(iii) sense of identity over time;

(iv) sense of unity or of being one and the same person.

Among these features, the sense of activity was crucial for Jaspers, since through it perceptions, sensations, thoughts, feelings, and actions are "personalized." The experience of one's mental acts as not being one's own, e.g. as alien or automatic, was termed "depersonalization" by Jaspers. Later editions of Jaspers's *General Psychopathology* were increasingly influenced by Kurt Schneider (Fuchs, 2013b). Jaspers now put the sense of activity in first place and further divided it into:

(i) Awareness of existence or of being-there (*Existenz-* or *Daseinsbewusstsein*), whose disturbance meant a self-alienation in different degrees.

(ii) Awareness of agency (*Vollzugsbewusstsein*), whose disturbance was now equivalent to experiencing one's thoughts or actions as being made, controlled, or drawn from outside.

On this basis, Kurt Schneider later coined the term "Ich-Störungen" (ego-disorders) for the schizophrenic experience of one's thoughts, actions, feelings, or bodily sensations being influenced or manipulated by others. In the first edition of *Clinical Psychopathology* (Schneider, 1950), since the notion of agency could hardly be attributed to feelings and spontaneous thoughts, he substituted the sense of activity by the term "mineness" (*Meinhaftigkeit*).

Two basic and closely related aspects of minimal self-awareness are self-ownership and self-agency. Self-ownership is the pre-reflexive sense that I am the one who is undergoing an experience. Self-agency is the pre-reflexive sense that I am the one who is initiating an action. The immediate awareness of the subjectivity of my experience or action involves that these are in some sense owned and generated by myself. These are the basic components of the experienced differentiation between self and non-self, my self and the object I perceive, and my representation of that object and the object itself.

Otherness

With "otherness" in this context we mean the experience a person has of other people. The way a person experiences other persons is obviously a cornerstone of her life-world.

In general terms, there is no "I" taken in itself, since we are always placed in a relation with the Other. The "I" is originally and ontologically relational. The Other may appear as a "You" or as an "It." The way the Other appears to me deeply affects not only the mode in which I experience him, but also the mode in which I experience myself in his presence. The "I" of the "I–You" combination is different from the "I" of the "I–It" combination. When a person says "I" he refers to one or other of these. In the personal relation an "I" confronts a "You." In the connection with things an "I" connects with an "It." These two attitudes constitute respectively the world of the "You" and the world of "It" (Buber, 1958). The other person as a "You" cannot be appropriated. So long as the "I" remains in the relationship with the "You" it cannot be reduced to an experienced object – an "It."

What distinguishes these two modes is not the object per se. We can relate to an object (say, the moon) as to a "You" (as for instance children and poets do), or to a person as to a thing. What changes is our attitude, not the object. This change of attitude may occur across time, as in one moment we may address a person as a "You" (for instance, in the "openness" of the therapeutic interview) or as an "It" (for instance, in the course of an assessment interview).

This account of the "I–You world" can be expanded in such a way as to capture the ontological implications of establishing an "I–You" relation in the therapeutic setting (Stanghellini, 2016b). Treating the Other as a "You" is not simply instrumental to establishing a better kind of relation in ethical or epistemological terms. Rather, it may generate a profound transformation of the basic structures of the life-world in which both the "I" (the therapist) and the "You" (the patient) live.

The majority of everyday relations are based on the immediate and pre-reflective face-to-face encounter with other persons, whose mental states (emotions, beliefs, desires, etc.) are expressed directly in their actions and are typically grasped as meaningful in this emergent, pragmatic context. In short, we are in touch with each other, first and foremost, through a direct contact or a fine pre-thematic attunement with the expressive behavior of other people. This pre-thematic attunement with the Other's behavior is grounded in one's emotional life.

The Other's behavior (postures, gestures, expressed emotions, gazes, and goal-oriented actions) intrinsically possesses an *expressive unity* (Scheler, 1973) and meaningfulness that we can directly grasp during the encounters, without any reflexive/introspective mediation. On this view the basic form of intersubjectivity is a particular kind of perception, thought to be innate: the newborn, it seems, is immediately able to respond to gestures and, from a very early age, can discriminate humans from inanimate objects (Johnson, 2000).

The perceptual understanding of others displays two main features: those of being *enacted* and fully *embodied*. The experience I have of other persons is *enactive* in the sense that it unfolds in a pragmatic and semantically meaningful, situational context that is a constitutive part of the encounter itself. Our relationships are given in a world that is, from the beginning, a shared world of action. Understanding other persons is fully *embodied* in the sense of being based on the resonance between my body and the Other's body, with the other given in his "expressive bodily presence" (Gallagher and Zahavi, 2012). From birth intersubjectivity is a sensorimotor, proprioceptive, and emotion-based apprehension of Others. Mother and infant create a pre-verbal communication context based on affective attunement. This implicit code – which develops hand in hand with a basic sense of self – is procedural, non-symbolic, and pre-reflective (Ammaniti and Gallese, 2014).

The role of the lived body or body-subject (the pre-reflective, implicit experience of the body) is of fundamental importance. The body-subject structures the primordial sense of self, grounds our natural immersion in the world, and organizes the immediate (sensorimotor) experience of the others as well as the attunement-cum-demarcation of self with other. In this perspective, my apprehension of the Other is first and foremost *intercorporeality*. This implies that my apprehension of the Other is inescapably rooted in the domain of my emotional life. The capacity to feel my emotions and to resonate with those of Others is the condition of possibility for my experience to be engaged in a social world. Needless to say my own emotions affect the way I experience and represent the Other.

An emphasis on intercorporeality is not meant to downplay the relevance of cognition (language, concepts, and constructs) in the task of understanding other persons. In particular circumstances, e.g. when confronted with difficult or ambiguous situations when what we perceive does not match the supervening actions or expressions, we may adopt a cognitively charged, strategic, introspective approach, drawing inferences or hypothesizing imaginative (simulation) routines as in pretense play (Hutto, 2013).

Such a form of intersubjectivity serves to represent mental states, and it may well depend on neurocognitive capacities such as working memory and inhibitory control, language and narrative competency, previous experience including semantic and episodic memory, personal history, and ethical arrangement of values. A central role is played by our *narrative competency* (Hutto, 2007), given that actions or expressions become intelligible when they are organized in a "narrative frame." In other words, full comprehension of an Other's behavior may require us to arrange what we see and perceive in a sort of story, continuously being updated. Using linguistic resources we achieve a "narrative framing" of the Other's behavior. Our commonsensical comprehension of Others is enriched by a large, culturally grounded database of *shared narratives* that depict mental states such as intentions and emotions.

In short: my experience of the Other emerges as a complex phenomenon, multi-dimensional or multi-faceted in its very nature. Intersubjectivity may sometimes work like a mirror, when my body implicitly and involuntarily echoes the Other's actions in order intuitively to grasp their meaning by re-enacting them. But also, at times, like a computational device: when I need to set the Other's actions in a linguistic-narrative framework in order to infer their meaning. In our everyday transactions we adopt all the modalities of intersubjectivity, privileging one or the other in accordance with the unfolding of the situation. The modalities of intersubjectivity (including their neural substrates) are not separate systems but fully integrated and continuously interacting. But in order to function appropriately, both systems – the intuitive and the computational – need to be attuned to the present situation, thus embedded in a temporal context matched and synchronized with that of the other person or persons with whom one interacts.

The ability to understand other persons is not equally distributed among people and the arrangement of intersubjective resources may vary from person to person: one person may be more reliant on *perceptive* and another more on *cognitive* resources. A cognitive-inferential approach may be endorsed as a coping strategy with respect to less developed perceptive-intuitive abilities (Ballerini, 2016).

7

An Example of Life-World Analysis

The exploration of patients' life-worlds involves at least two distinct steps. The first – called *phenomenal exploration* – is the gathering of qualitative descriptions of the lived experiences about the patient. As lived experiences are always situated within the grounds of body, self, time, space, and others, we adopt these basic dimensions of lived experience to organize the data. In order to investigate these dimensions, the inquiry will start with questions such as:

(1) How does the patient experience his world? How does he or she express, move, and define space as an embodied subject?

(2) What is the patient's experience of existential time? Is there a sense of continuity over time, or are there breaks of self-awareness?

(3) Does the patient feel effective as an agent in the world, or rather as being exposed to the world?

(4) Is there a tendency to take an external perspective to one's body, actions, and self? Do the knowing and the feeling subject coincide or diverge?

(5) How is the patient's ability to empathize with others, to take their perspective? How does he/she experience his/her relationships? (adapted from Fuchs, 2010).

The result will be a rich and detailed collection of the patient's self-descriptions related to each dimension, for example, temporal continuity/discontinuity, space flat/filled with saliences, bodily coherence/fragmentation, self–world demarcation/permeability, self–other attunement/disattunement, and so on. In this way, using first-person accounts, we detect the critical points where the constitution of experience and action is vulnerable and open to derailments.

The second step implies a shift to phenomenology proper that seeks the basic structures or existential dimensions of the life-worlds the patient lives in. Any phenomenon is viewed as the expression of a given form of human subjectivity; abnormal phenomena are the outcome of a more or less profound modification of human subjectivity. Phenomenology is committed to attempting to discover a common source that ties the seemingly heterogeneous phenomena together, from which we can make sense of the relevant lived experience. This is done by finding similarities among the manifold phenomena and, possibly, the deep or structural change in the form of experience/action related to that specific existential dimension (spatiality, temporality, embodiment, and so on) that would offer an explanation for the various changes that occur in the patients. Section 2 of this book contains the most relevant examples of this in the realm of severe mental disorders. For example, in schizophrenia, the person may lose his or her anchoring in the lived body as a *Gestalt* of organs and functions delimited from the external environment (Stanghellini, Ballerini, et al., 2012),

Table 7.1 Prompts for life-world exploration: experience of other persons in schizophrenia patients (from ARS-2.0)

General questions	Can you tell me how much time you spent with other persons in the last three months? What sort of things have you been doing with them? Can you describe these in great detail? What does it mean for you to be with the others? Which emotions or thoughts do you feel when you are with them? Do you have any idea about what the others think or feel? Do you feel like the others?
Questions addressing specific domains of intersubjectivity	Do you feel a sort of detachment from other persons? Do they appear somehow unnatural? Do you happen to feel distant from the others? Or as if a barrier is in between you? Do you happen not to be able to understand the intentions of the others? Or the rules of the context you are in? Does it happen to you that you need to reduce your social contacts because the others are somehow enigmatic? Did someone tell you that your behavior was inadequate to circumstances? Did you ever have the feeling of being radically different from all the other persons? Or that there is something non-human in yourself? Or to be of another race, or from another planet? If so, what makes you think this? Did you ever feel yourself to be at the mercy of others? Or to be at the center of the others' attention? Or that things happen exactly because you are there, that they happen *for* you? How can you explain these sensations? Have you had the feeling of being without barriers? Or as if you were melting with the others? Or as if the others could invade you? Or transparent?

or in temporal continuity (Fuchs, 2013a), or in anisotropic space, meaning space that is imbued with a point of view (Sass and Pienkos, 2013b), or in intersubjective attunement and common sense (Stanghellini and Ballerini, 2011), or in selfhood (Stanghellini, 2013b) (Table 7.1).

We will give here an example of the *process* of the therapeutic interview guided by the hermeneutic-phenomenological framework. Imagine you are interviewing a patient (let's call him Giacomo) who tells you this story:

Enter a garden with plants, herbs, and flowers. It can be as lovely as you like. It can be the mildest season of the year. In every part you look you will find suffering. The whole vegetable family is in a state of souffrance to some degree. Here a rose is injured by the sun that gave it life; it wrinkles, languishes, wilts. There a lily is cruelly sucked by a bee in its most sensitive, vital parts.[1]

The first thing you may think is that this is not what could happen to anyone entering a garden which is apparently flourishing and gorgeous. You ask yourself "What makes a flourishing garden turn into a real hell?"

This question, on the *condition of possibility* of this type of experience, makes you turn your attention, rather than to symptoms or pathogenetic mechanisms, to this person's first-personal experience, and more specifically to the way Giacomo approaches the garden as a significant or emblematic part of his life-world. In order to attain a faithful description of his life-world you need to obtain information about the way he lives space, time, and the materiality of things in this scenario. Of special relevance is lived distance as the key feature of the spatial structure – the relation between man and things in space.

You (the interviewer) at this moment try to imagine what the experience of space is like for Giacomo. During the therapeutic interview you perform *imaginative variations* through which you try to focus the essential character of the phenomenon in question. Your imagination brings you to feel that Giacomo experiences an *excessive nearness* of things that makes him "see" on the surface of things what would be normally invisible. Such lack of distance between Giacomo and the surrounding world is part of the metamorphosis of lived space: lack of distance between Giacomo and the garden implies that he does not have a panoramic view but that he can only see fragments of it. Also, the lack of distance implies that each entity, either an animal or plant, is perceived as attacked, surrounded, besieged. This extreme proximity to things also entails a metamorphosis of materiality – the way things appear to the person. Plants, in the mildest season of the year, are in a state of *souffrance*, a bee turns into an insect that cruelly penetrates and sucks, and even the sun, the first source of life for our planet, becomes an oppressor. Lived time is also involved in this metamorphosis of the life-world: things are not perceived as stable; instead they conceal ultra-rapid biological processes which cause *decay*.

The therapeutic interview is a circle or continuous flipping between the analysis of the individual person's subjective experiences and the background of *theoretical knowledge* that may help to make sense of it. One step is the active bracketing of all previous knowledge and beliefs about a given type of phenomenon that may distort with its prejudices the understanding of that individual phenomenon. Another step consists in contrasting this "free" understanding of that individual phenomenon with a family of legitimate preconceptions which by analogy may help shed light on the phenomenon in question. The progressive clarification of an individual case always implies a pre-comprehension, that is, something which is originally given and waits to be better articulated in the hermeneutical circle by means of contrasting it with an insight into the individual case itself.

---

[1] Giacomo Leopardi (1992: 4175). This is not in fact a patient's narrative, but a passage from *Zibaldone*, a work by Giacomo Leopardi, one of Italy's most influential poets during the eary nineteenth century. Leopardi's philosophy is commonly considered pessimistic: in fact, what really matters to the poet is *objectivity*. By no means do we intend to demonstrate that Leopardi was affected by some form of mental disorder, such as obsessive compulsive disorder, or contamination obsession. We only use this piece from his notebooks as the starting point of an example of life-world analysis.

Hence, what you have learnt from Giacomo makes you remember that once you read an essay by Erwin Straus (1948) on obsessive phenomena and that his attempts to make sense of the metamorphosis of the life-world you have observed in Giacomo is relevant for your understanding of Giacomo's perceptions. Straus takes into consideration three clinical varieties of obsessions: compulsive neurosis, obsessive psychosis concerned with contamination, and a third group characterized by "worries." The patients from the first group experience the impulse of fighting against their own instincts, most of which are recognized as morally inadmissible. Contamination obsessions are characterized by a never-ending fight against "decay," experienced as both a cosmic power and substance. Contamination cases according to Straus typically develop into psychosis. The third group is intermediate but somewhat closer to the contamination subtype.

You are not primarily interested in the diagnosis that you could make guided by Straus's analyses. Rather, you want to understand what it is like to live in such a world that makes Giacomo experience a garden in spring as a hell of decay and fight for survival. You have in mind that all investigations on subjectivity have to pay preliminary attention to deciding which characteristics should be considered fundamental for a correct understanding of human beings and their relation to the world. Following Heidegger (1927/1962) you know that lived experiences are always situated within the ground of *existentialia* – the basic structures of subjectivity within which each single experience is situated – and only if these grounds are described experientially is it possible to develop a first-person, descriptive psychopathology in which human experience is the central focus (Pollio, Henley, and Thompson, 1997). These "forms" of human experience are neither the causes of certain symptoms, nor their psychological motivations; rather, they serve as the guidelines to describe the mode in which consciousness is configured in order to experience things in a given way. It is important to highlight that at this point of the interview there is a move from understanding conceived as the interviewer's reliving the patient's experience (as it was in the tradition emphasizing the importance of empathy), to the understanding of that patient as being situated in his world. Following these guidelines, you start exploring in great detail the life-world of this person (a previous analysis can be found in Stanghellini and Muscelli, 2007).

Lived Time

Lived time is the way each person experiences time. Cosmic objective time and the subjective experience of time do not coincide. The latter is not homogeneous, e.g. youth and health diminish distance between present and future, whereas old age and fatigue expand it (Straus, 1948). Essential aspects of personal experience of time are for instance change/continuity (our experience of becoming over time), limits/choices (how we cope with limited amounts of time), and fast/slow (the *tempo* of our doings and experiencing).

Many authors agree upon the general idea of a lived time blockage in obsessive-compulsive disorder (Minkowski, 1933/1970; von Gebsattel, 1938; Straus, 1948). If the current of time stops, the person is trapped in the eternal fight against the irregular and decaying world. It is because lived time has come to a standstill that things begin to decompose. Stagnation and putrefaction are two facets of the same coin. Other authors suggest that persons with obsessions mistrust the natural flow of things, and are in constant need to control this flow (Fenichel, 1945). They may experience reality as a constant, fleeting flow that refuses to be pinned down (Ingram, 1979).

Lived Space

Lived space is primarily a lived distance which "binds me to the things which count and exist for me, and links them to each other. This distance measures the scope of my life at every moment" (Merleau-Ponty, 1945/1962: 286). We are not referring to distance as a geometric unit: lived distance is referred to as the lived space that connects a person to his environment. In fact, it is the modulation of the lived distance that allows man to interact with his world or, in a given case, to defend himself from the "aggression" of a threatening world. A "homely" lived space is characterized by a balanced relation between distance and proximity, where one is able to keep things "at hand" but not too close. Too much closeness would mean the impossibility of utilizing objects and would soon turn into an impediment. In Merleau-Ponty's words: "Sometimes between myself and the events there is a certain amount of play (*Spielraum*), which ensures that my freedom is preserved while the events do not cease to concern me. Sometimes, on the other hand, the lived distance is both too small and too great; the majority of the events cease to count for me, while the nearest ones obsess me. They enshroud me like the night and rob me of my individuality and freedom. I can literally no longer breathe; I am possessed" (1945/1962: 286).

Lived space for Giacomo is confinement, restriction, annihilation. The need for a shrinking space emerges from the obligation to avoid contamination: there is a correlation between the amount of effort put in trying to avoid contamination and the limitation of space.

Materiality

Materiality expresses the idea of a linkage between things, their qualities and man's emotional attitude to them (Straus, 1948). The form of the matter is named by Straus "physiognomic": it is the appearance of the world as a physical entity; a certain physiognomy is always co-given with a corresponding emotional reaction (e.g. decay and disgust). "Physiognomic" means matter's exterior and the corresponding human emotional feeling. For these reasons the "physiognomic" is a descriptive term useful to a better comprehension of man's relation to his environment.[2]

The physiognomy of things for Giacomo is characterized by fragmentation and decay, and the corresponding emotion is *disgust* (Phillips et al., 1997, 1998). To Giacomo, matter in the garden has lost its unity: it is constantly decaying, dying, in the process of decomposing. This phenomenon is related to an original stagnation of time, whose physiognomy is that of rottenness and putrefaction (von Gebsattel, 1938; Ballerini and Stanghellini, 1989). It is a world in which everything appears without a neat shape. Such matter is accompanied by repulsion and disgust.

In this alternation between the attention to the individual case of Giacomo and your glances to the "background knowledge" that characterizes the hermeneutic in the therapeutic interview, you remember that once you came across an essay by Ludwig Binswanger, "The case of Lola Voss" (1928/1963), describing a case of contamination obsession turning

---

[2] Physiognomic characters are always determined by social and cultural factors: today's theoretical attitude towards things is dominated by the scientific approach which reduces everything to objects, and objects to "samples." Since science cannot consider the emotional relation to matter, through the scientific approach worldly things lose the complexity of their physiognomy and are transformed into objects far different from what we really and mostly experience in our everyday life.

into a full-blown psychosis. Lived space in Lola's world is altered: things are too close to each other and this proximity is the origin of their being lived as evil. As time is discontinuous, being shaped by the momentary presence of the Terrible, of what she fears in a moment, space too is discontinuous being organized around "infectious focuses." Lola interprets everything on the basis of spatial vicinity: objects pass their terrifying qualities on to what is next to them. Lola cannot keep things at a distance. Sometimes she tries to artificially enlarge space by closing her eyes, to keep the contagion of things away from her. The ultimate consequence is that she does not inhabit space, but she must "read" space: she is compelled to interpret space according to magic, oracular rules (e.g. she endlessly looks for "signs" to sort out what can be touched and what cannot be touched) to save herself from the contagion of things.

Binswanger's essay evokes in your mind a paper by Lorenzo Calvi (2005) who, in a similar vein, reports:

> Between the surface of the body and that of objects, in the place where they consume each other, there is a category of invisible and omnipresent things, jumping from one surface to the other and being absolutely ungraspable. Nobody has seen germs but, if they truly exist, they clearly demonstrate there are things which are mobile, unreliable, unsafe, although they could pretend to be inoffensive. *Nobody can really demonstrate that all this is not true for all things.* (Calvi, 2005: 92; our translation and italics)

By means of an experiment of imagination, you realize that an essential feature of human experience (including your own experience) is that distant things in a landscape are more beautiful and desirable than proximate ones. By consequence, pleasure will grow or diminish according to the growth or decrease of distance between the person and the world. A close approach to things is necessary to the understanding of reality but it also brings suffering. To reduce the distance from anything in the world does not reveal death; rather, reduction lets violence and suffering appear. What is brought out through the approximation to things is the disintegration operated by violent natural agents. Accordingly, if imagination is inhibited by proximity to things, pleasure is gradually restrained and turns into suffering. In the end, pleasure and suffering depend on distance.

Giacomo's Life-World

With all this in place, you now try to grasp the overall structure of Giacomo's experience. First of all, Giacomo feels that space is growing smaller, that things are getting too close. The reduction of lived distance, that getting very close to things, has three foremost effects:

(1) *Things are too near to the person.* This has three main consequences:

   (a) Because of their extreme vicinity, *things are experienced as not manageable.* They cannot be handled in normal ways. This helps you to make sense of some otherwise "crazy" behaviors of this person. As an example: Giacomo may state that he cannot wear anymore the clothes he was wearing the day he paid the visit to the garden because they are "stained by death," or that all objects or situations that are connected to the date (say it was mid-April) on which he was in the garden are also contaminated by the atmosphere of decay (for instance, he cannot take a pill whose dosage is 25 mg, or buy a good that costs 2 or 5 euros, or a multiple of these). These behaviors, which psychopathology labels as "compulsions," include magic rituals to create distance and separate objects one from another in order to reduce the possibility of reciprocal contamination between these objects. In spatial terms, compulsions related to contamination obsessions can be seen as a strenuous endeavor to organize one's space (Segrott and Doell, 2004). All that appears irrational is actually the attempt at regaining control over one's everyday environment.

(b) Extreme proximity incurs *the loss of the experience of the object's entirety*. If we were asked to provide an example about the decrease of distance and its consequences, we might think of what happens when we enjoy a beautiful landscape. When we look at the entire landscape, we are able to see from the sky to the mountain tops, from the clouds to the grassy valleys, we can take pleasure in the view, and the landscape itself seems a perfectly harmonic whole. If an obstacle or any other obstruction impeded the view of even just a small part of the entire landscape, we would not sense the same beauty: one detail can contribute to the creation of a beautiful landscape but cannot arouse any sense of beauty. The sense of beauty, as well as meaningfulness, find their origin in completeness, entirety, unity. Loss of entirety here means that things are not seen as a whole: it has no more beauty, no meaning, no functionality. Its sense is lost. Although his perception of reality may seem much more detailed than what happens normally, Giacomo is apparently unable to see completeness. This helps understand that his concern with details is not a ritual or a compulsion. He does not see whole things: he focuses on portions, parts, details. His world has lost its unity, things are not integrated in one environment, everything is fragmented, and fragments attain greater importance than the whole. Entirety is replaced by the un-form, or *aneidos* as Straus names it.

(c) The third effect is the *emergence of the microscopic* dimension of things. Things, that cannot appear as a whole, appear as they would appear in a microscope: polluted with insects and microbes (which literally means forms of life of minute dimensions). Obviously, this is not real perception of microbes, rather a concretistic representation of the fleeting, occult, uncontrollable, and menacing nature of what goes on inside things. The reduction of lived distance reveals to the gaze of the person with contamination obsessions the microscopic life, which is unperceivable from a distance. The essential outcome of the microscopic approach is a simultaneous loss of significance and the finding of the biological aspect in anything. In fact, the microscopic view notices the invisible processes of material, physical, biological transformation, sees the minuscule and complex life on any surface, becomes aware of the imperceptible life that goes on even though unseen. The corollary of the microscopic approach is that the process of decomposition is seen to be active everywhere. What was stability and steadiness now is endless alteration and uncontrollable decay. Life should appear and be felt as a whole, something that "naturally" happens, and not as the result of a multitude of microscopic processes.

Compulsions are necessary in relation to the nature of this microscopic space that causes things to be as if they were living beings. Objects are turned into subjects: they move as if they were alive (subject to decay). Giacomo's experience is permanently altered by the emotion of *disgust*: this emotion is related to matter, which has lost its functional, aesthetic, and economic value. Matter is just repulsive. Things are not unified and organic, but substances in the process of decay, eternally perishing. This attribute pervades the entire reality and forces the obsessive person to relentlessly try to free herself from the corresponding disgust.

(2) *Space between things is too small.* Contamination can be extremely fast thanks to the microscopic quality of the space: any contaminated thing can pass the contamination over to other things. The outcome is that this process of contamination is "accelerating." Acceleration, another essential attribute of this person's lived world, regards both extension of contamination and intensity of psychological suffering. Space in which everything accelerates becomes a frightening chaos, unless a ritual manages the purification. This system of disorder must be opposed systematically. Order, established through rituals that become compulsive, would impede contamination. Therefore, it is crucial to organize a space where things cannot circulate freely. Even when the circulation is commenced by someone else, a well-organized space would end the movement, slow down the dangerous run. Borders, limited areas, confines: these are the spatial elements contrasting contamination, since they can bring things to a halt.

(3) *The remaining space grows to infinity.* Giacomo's extreme approximation to things renders space immense. His interest in the smallest things makes the amount of space virtually infinite. Elements are magnified if we approach them; by consequence their dimension, the space they occupy, gets bigger. The closer we get to an object, the bigger its space gets. An example of this phenomenon is what everyone experiences when working on a drawing, a computer aided design or any other work of precision: we tend to magnify single small parts to make them perfect, and we do not proceed with the work until we get those done (even if we know the imperfection will not even be visible in the final result or noticed by anyone). Eventually, the dimension of the work will be much bigger than what it should actually be. One could see in this attitude also a moral component: this person cannot do anything else unless the imperfection is solved. This could explain also the association between the transformation of the life-world into a contaminating space and a sense of guilt.

In short: Giacomo lives in a *counter-world* whose major feature is the breakdown of the meaningful *Gestalt* of a gorgeous garden into a series of microscopic details that make the grass appear as the chaotic space where each fragment struggles for life. Accordingly, microscopic aspects of reality emerge to visibility and things develop into vehicles for microscopic life which otherwise would stay unknown. Inanimate objects are "biologized": life is perceived where and when it should not be. This microscopic distance gives shape to his world: space, time, and materiality depend on the excessive nearness of things to the person. Paradoxically, this closeness to things renders the world immense. In such a threatening enormous world, contamination can be so rapid because distance between things is small. Spatial order is characterized by "contiguity": anything is contiguous to anything else (and to the person too). Germs can rapidly invade such a space because there is no distance to cover. Subsequently, the endless and despairing effort of this person will be to redefine confines and distances. This seems to be Giacomo's pragmatic motive: separating, isolating, since the only obstacle to contamination would be space, but in this life-world space has no void distances, there is no empty space. Also, he needs to have an "objective" look at the garden, perhaps in order to defend himself from the atmosphere of decay. Through this "objective" stance the garden does not appear as the realm of life, but that of impending death. Yet, Giacomo's "objective" attitude contributes to fragmentation, loss of common-sense meaningfulness, disgust and decay. Also, a key character of lived time in such a world is "acceleration." Things are not perceived as stable; instead they conceal rapid biological processes which cause decay. There is a sort of *vibration* in any substance. All matter, even things that should be seen as just "tools," becomes "organic" because it is seen as if through a microscope. Under the action of microscopic beings matter is ruined, decomposed, destroyed. The person cannot see the whole things but just the microscopic parts of those. His relation to the world is decided by the operation of separation: his perception disintegrates the unity of things and sees fractions of things. Anything is disgusting when separated from what it belongs to, when it loses the harmony of completeness. Disgust is the emotion that accompanies the separation of a detail from the whole. All these parts coming from the disintegration of things become waste, disgusting bits and pieces. We are disgusted by the physiognomy of decay, whose central characteristic is the separation of parts or details from the integrity of the whole, or the *aneidos* – literally the un-form:

> Curls on a head look lovely and attractive, but the same hair found in the soup is disgusting; perhaps we should like to cut one of these curls as a souvenir, but we should be disgusted to collect the hair left in a comb. Saliva spit out is disgusting, an expression of our contempt, but on fresh lips and tongue the saliva is not disgusting. Separation from the integrity of the living organism indicates a transition to death; it signifies decay, the process of decomposition, then again the dead. (Straus, 1948: 13)

8 What Are Emotions and Why Are They Relevant to the Therapeutic Interview?

The fundamental way of being situated in the world is being in a given feeling-state or emotional tonality. Emotions are the primordial medium in which I encounter the world as a set of affordances: a set of relevant possibilities that are my own possibilities as a person situated in this particular world. This being situated in a world of possibilities through a certain feeling is called *Befindlichkeit* (Heidegger, 1927/1962) – a term that combines the notion of location (finding oneself somewhere) and that of being in a certain feeling-state (*Stimmung*). The concept of *Befindlichkeit* focuses on the set of affordable actions of a person who is located in a certain context and affected by a certain emotion that allows him to see the things that surround him as disclosing certain (and not other) possibilities. The significance of an event or state of affairs is not merely a matter of its intrinsic properties, but rather of its relation to me and my current emotional engagement.

The main force of the concept of *Befindlichkeit* is that it emphasizes the work of emotions as an uncovering (*Erschlossenheit*) of one's situatedness in the world, instead of an impediment to objectively appreciating a certain state of things. Emotions are not merely *passions* of the mind that get in the way of rational thinking and action. Rather, they are the key for a person's self-understanding in a given situation. This means that the analysis of a person's emotions is the *via regia* for understanding this person. Emotions reveal how the world is *for me*. The concept of *Befindlichkeit* is closely tied to that of "understanding." We can only understand ourselves and the world in which we are situated through the context of our practical engagement, and this engagement is primordially enveloped in a certain emotion. This way of looking at emotions has fundamental implications for care that will be best appreciated if we first discuss the rapport between feelings and emotions and that between moods and affects.

Feelings and Emotions

Emotions are kinetic, dynamic forces that drive us in our ongoing interactions with the environment. This definition of "emotion" focuses on the *embodied* nature of emotions. From this vantage, emotions are basically "bioregulatory reactions that aim at promoting, directly or indirectly, the sort of physiological states that secure not just survival but survival regulated into the range that we, conscious and thinking creatures, identify with well-being" (Damasio, 2004: 50; for similar accounts, see Russell, 2003; Panksepp, 2005a, 2005b). A closer analysis of Damasio's account will help us to see why they cannot be simply reduced to biological adaptive reactions.

There is a close resemblance between an emotion (emotion comes from Latin *ex movere*, that is, what makes us move, the origin of movement) as the embodied motivation to move in a given way, and *intentionality* – a force that directs and connects (*Gerichtetsein*, Husserl,

2002) to reality. Emotions can be understood as *embodied intentionality*. They provide my orientation in the life-world. Emotions orient my movement and my receptivity. They make me turn my attention in a given direction, to be absorbed by a more or less defined object, to move (or move away) in a given direction.

This definition of "emotion" focuses on the embodied nature of emotions, but rejects the reduction of the person to a biological mechanism (like visceral changes mediated by the autonomic nervous system). When I experience a given emotion, say anger, I as a human person am not compelled to act in a hostile way. As a human person, I can decide whether to behave aggressively or not, to evaluate whether my anger is good or bad, and finally to use my angry feelings as a means to understand myself in the situation in which I am engaged. In short: I am not just passive with respect to my emotions. I can voluntarily relate myself to my emotions. My personhood is constituted by my active relation to my *Befindlichkeit*, that is, to my being situated by my emotions.

This definition also rejects the conceptualization of emotions as pure "mental" or disembodied phenomena because an emotion is not a purely and primarily cognitive phenomenon affecting the mind, but a phenomenon rooted in one's lived body, and it can to a certain extent be pre-cognitive and subconscious (Panksepp, 2005a; Prinz, 2005). Emotions are primarily embodied phenomena since they are characterized by their connection to motivation and movement. Emotions are bodily functional states, which motivate and may produce movements. This view is held by contemporary evolutionary psychologists (Plutchik, 1980), as well as by phenomenological analysts (Sheets-Johnstone, 1999a, 1999b). As functional states that motivate movement, emotions are protential states in the sense that they project the person into the future providing a felt readiness for action (Gallagher, 2005).

Feelings are an inherent part of all emotional experience. Feeling is the *what-it-is-like* or experiential dimension of being in a given emotional state. That is to say that each emotion has (at least) two components: its biological pre-phenomenal mechanism and its phenomenal feeling. Although how an emotion feels may remain vague to the person, feelings are essential to recognize a given emotion.

The feeling dimension of emotion is what permits us to distinguish emotions among other psychic phenomena (perception, deliberation, evaluation, judging, etc.). Emotions immerse the other cognitive functions in their non-rational movement whenever they appear.

Feelings are also crucial for differentiating between different kinds of emotional experiences, since we are not aware of the biological processes inherent in our emotions (e.g. the release of epinephrine) but only of the feelings that accompany them (e.g. increased heart rate and readiness for fight or flight).

One further reason why the feeling dimension of emotion is important is because emotions can be both conscious and subconscious. Conscious emotions take up, by virtue of their intentional attitude, a substantial part of our attention in a given situation. For example, I choose not to undress myself in front of other people because I feel ashamed. Subconscious emotions, on the contrary, are not direct objects in our attentional field. They manifest themselves through certain feelings. Usually these feelings are vague and opaque (as in the case of moods; see below). However, the feelings of an emotion are an essential component of the emotion itself and we, as persons, need to acknowledge these feelings to fully access the emotion. We will give detailed descriptions of "bad moods" (e.g. dysphoria, boredom, etc.) in the second part of this volume.

Furthermore, the constellation of feelings involved in an emotional experience may contain more or less explicit cognitive elements. The feelings involved in fear, for example, may tend to block our higher cognitive skills to promote the immediate instinct to flee from the object that causes the emotion. In sadness, feelings and cognition are intrinsically intertwined. The feelings are both subject and object for our reflections. We are sad because we feel sad, but the thought involved in our sadness may enhance or diminish our feeling of sadness (LeDoux, 2000).

To access these emotional states, we need to pay attention to the diffuse and vague constellation of feelings involved in our interaction with the world. This is indeed a difficult task. Nevertheless, we believe that by sorting out the main characteristics of the different feelings involved in emotional states we gain an effective tool to develop an understanding of how someone lives, experiences, and understands himself as an embodied and situated person. One way to access and articulate emotional experiences is describing each emotion in terms of the *choreography* it implies. Once we understand emotions as embodied motivation for moving in a given way, we can easily see that each emotion designs its own choreography. Choreography literally means "dance-writing": it is the discipline that describes the sequences of bodily movements in a given scenario. Each choreography includes the design of the movements of a person (a dancer), and of the design of the environment (the scenario) in which these movements are situated.

Indeed, it is helpful to ask patients to portray their emotions in terms of their choreography. As emotional feelings are sometimes not easy to express, especially in purely cognitive terms, having in mind the choreographies of emotions may help the interviewer to assist the patient to provide a reliable description of the emotion she is experiencing. We will give some examples of choreographies of emotions (Smith, 1986) as guidelines for the therapeutic interview.

A *sad* person will describe her emotion as the feeling of flowing downwards in a slow, sinking manner, while at the same time things around appear to her to be forlornly sinking and sagging downwards.

A person affected by *joy* will say that she feels herself flowing upwards in a radiating manner while things around her have an uplifted momentum too.

In *pride* I feel I'm going upwards, as an inflated rising, while things around me become little as compared to me.

In *humiliation* I flow downwards in a plummeting, quick and violent drop, while persons around me get bigger and look at me.

In retaliatory *anger*, I feel driven forwards, violently attacking, while the "object" of anger gets big and occupies the foreground.

In *love*, I flow forwards in a gently binding way, while the loved one flows forwards, towards me.

In *repugnance*, I flow backwards creating a centripetal vortex, while things flow forward, attracted towards me by the vortex.

In *awe*, I flow backwards and downwards in a shuddering manner, while things flow forwards and upwards – towering above me.

In *fear*, I move backwards in a shrinking and cringing manner, while things flow forwards, towards me in a looming and menacing manner.

In *anxiety*, I feel suspended in a quavering manner over an inner bottomlessness, while the atmosphere, not things themselves, is felt as a menace.

In *anguish*, I feel constricted in a corner, while things, space itself, flow towards me in an oppressive manner.

What Emotions Are For: Engagement, Enactment, and Attunement

Emotions are not merely passions that affect the mind and hamper rational thinking and action. They are essential to situate a person in the world, that is, to establish and preserve one's vital contact with reality. Indeed, emotions contribute to establish:

- my feeling involved in the world (engagement);
- my grasping the meanings of worldly objects (enactment);
- my pre-reflexive understanding of others' actions (attunement).

Emotions and Engagement

Emotions make me feel the world as real. Without emotions, the world appears as unreal, devoid of any interest and existential meaning. The world is *simply there*, I am a mere spectator of its happenings. Reality does not affect me; all vital contact with it is lost. Without emotions, things that inhabit my lived space appear as mere *objects*, things that stand in front of me without any relation with the practical needs and desires of my own body (Scheler, 2008). I am not involved; the world out there is merely the object of my theoretical and disinterested gaze. I see things as a sum of *realia* which fill up the geometrical space and stand one next to the other just "proximally" – not as "equipment." I see objects devoid of their readiness-to-hand, nearly as geometric bodies distributed within a purely geometric space – exactly as in De Chirico's or Magritte's paintings.

Emotions and Enactment

Enaction means that knowledge is action-specific, i.e. situated and embodied (Varela, Thompson, and Rosch, 1991). Emotions provide the motivational background for action. They situate me in the world and circumscribe my possibilities for action. My body via my emotions *inhabits* the world, that is, it structures my possibilities to use things in view of my vital and existential needs. The meaning of something is the way we put it to use. The basic kind of knowledge we have of situations we encounter in the world is not merely theoretical cognition, but rather a kind of involvement, of emotion-laden concern which manipulates things and "puts them to use." Things in the world are encountered as *pragmata*, that is to say, that which one has to do with in one's "concernful dealings (praxis)" (Heidegger, 1927/ 1962). If and only if I am moved by emotions are things in the world *pragmata*, that is, something in-order-to. Another way to put this is saying that, thanks to emotions, things have *handles* (Scheler, 2008): they appear as *equipment*. Emotions organize my possibilities to grasp things as parts of a situation in which I am engaged. I literally *grasp* the meaning of one thing, since this meaning is exactly the specific manipulability (*Handlichkeit*) of one thing.

The absence of emotions brings about a radical transformation of the lived world whose main features are the abandonment of all existentially relative *handles* on things and a metamorphosis of lived space. If my emotion-based involvement in the world is switched off, my grasp on the world will fade away too. Things in the world will not immediately relate to my body as existentially relative utensils. They become non-utilizable, and as such meaningless. Things appear devoid of practical meanings – in a word: meaningless. Lived space grows homogeneous, isotropic (Sass and Pienkos, 2013b), that is, devoid of any salience or point of orientation.

Emotions and Attunement

Attunement is a pre-reflexive, pre-verbal, and tacit bridge linking the emotional lives of other persons with my own. Emotional attunement between my own and the Other's emotions provides the basis for intersubjectivity. My understanding of the Other's actions is based on my capacity to resonate with the other's emotions. Husserl uses the concept of *Paarung*, that is, the coupling of one flesh with another flesh (Husserl, 1950). The basis for intersubjectivity is the direct perception of the Other's emotional life: the immediate perceptive bond with the Other's body (Scheler, 1927/1973, 1973). Intersubjectivity is the *pathic* (emotional) identification with the other's body (Merleau-Ponty, 1945/1962).

Without this capacity for emotional resonance other people and the social world in general would appear mechanical and incomprehensible. If my own body is unable to emotionally resonate with the Other's body, then the Other is experienced as an automaton, an entity moved by some mechanical device rather than by her own emotions. The social world loses its characteristic as a network of relationships among bodies moved by emotions and turns into a cool, incomprehensible game, from which the person feels excluded, and whose meaning is sought through the discovery of abstract algorithms, the elaboration of impersonal rules (for details, see Chapter 14).

Moods and Affects

There are two kinds of emotions: affects and moods. Both moods and affects are characterized by the constellation of feelings involved in the experience of them, and an analysis of the phenomenology of these feelings enables a better understanding of their influence on the person. The distinction between moods and affects may seem a purely nominalistic querelle. It is, however, important not to conflate the two; we need two different concepts to address two different sets of phenomena.

An in-depth discussion of the concepts of "mood" and "affect" is scantily provided in textbooks of psychiatry and psychopathology. Textbooks (Tasman, Kay, and Lieberman, 1997; Stoudemire, 1998; Hales and Yudofsky, 1999; Kaplan and Sadock, 2005) primarily use two dimensions to define "mood" and contrast it to "affect": one is temporal, the other is internal versus external or subjective versus objective. Although the definitions we find in different textbooks are not consistent, generally "mood" is defined as sustained and internal, whereas "affect" is momentary and external (Hales, Yudofsky, and Tallbot, 1999). For instance, Kaplan and Sadock (2005) distinguish mood ("pervasive and sustained feeling tone that is experienced internally and that, in the extreme, can markedly influence virtually all aspects of a person's behaviour and perception of the world") from affect ("the external expression of the internal feeling tone"). Also, in the DSM, "mood" is contrasted with "affect" accordingly (although in a rather indirect manner): affect is "a pattern of observable behaviours that is the expression of subjectively experienced feeling state (emotion)," whereas mood is equated with "emotion." We can infer that, according to the DSM, mood is the experienced feeling-state that entails a configuration of observable comportments (affects). It is also said that in contrast with affect, which refers to more fluctuating changes in emotional "weather," mood refers to a more pervasive and sustained emotional "climate."

Phenomenology has contributed to explaining this distinction in an explicit and systematic way (Smith, 1986; Stanghellini and Rosfort, 2013b). This distinction is merely incipient in Husserl's writings and is made explicit by Scheler (1973), Heidegger (1927/1962), Sartre (1939), and Ricoeur (1950, 1960): whereas affects are responses to a phenomenon that is grasped as their motivation, moods do not possess such directedness to a motivating object. Although their terminology differs, often confusingly (Scheler, *Affekten/Gefühlen*; Heidegger, *Affekten/Stimmungen*; Sartre, *affects/emotions*; Ricoeur, *sentiments schematisés/sentiments informes*), their analyses of the phenomena concur in the general characteristics. Affects are focused, intentional, and possess directedness. Affects are felt as motivated; they are more determinate than moods and more articulated. Affects do not open up a horizontal awareness, but occupy all my attentional space (e.g. in fear I am completely absorbed by the phenomenon that terrifies me). When I am affected, a relevant feature of the world captivates me, irrupts into my field of awareness without me having decided to turn my attention to it. I become spellbound to it and all my attention is captured by it. Typical examples of captivating affects are grief (when the death of a beloved person occupies all my attentional space) or phobias.

Moods, on the contrary, are unfocused and non-intentional. They do not possess directedness and aboutness. They are felt as unmotivated, and there are no "felt causes" for them. They are more indefinite and indeterminate than affects and are often inarticulate. Moods have a horizontal absorption in the sense that they attend to the world as a whole, not focusing on any particular object or situation. Moods often manifest themselves as prolonged feeling-states as opposed to the more instantaneous nature of affect. Whereas most affects fill up the whole field of awareness for a brief period (e.g. in fear or anger), moods convey a constellation of vague feelings that permeate my whole field of awareness, and they often last for a longer period than affects.

Moods are global feeling-states that do not focus on any specific object in my field of awareness. When we are in a certain mood we relate ourselves to the world and to ourselves through that mood. In euphoria, the perception of my body is feeble and may even vanish. I feel absorbed in my concerns; my self-awareness, my body, and the world fuse together in perfect harmony. In sadness, the perception of my body comes to the foreground.

I may feel my body as an obstacle, a hindrance separating me from the world and perhaps even from myself. Thus, moods are atmospheric and often corporeal in that they permeate my perception of the environment. They can bring me closer to or distance me from the world in that they elicit a certain atmosphere that becomes the tonality through which I perceive the world and myself. When I am feeling happy, the world and other persons appear in a soft light of possibility and openness; I feel differently from when I am jealous. In this case, things appear as prowling perils; even the most sincere smile might be perceived as false and dangerous to my person.

An important aspect of moods is that in virtue of being prolonged and pervasive feeling-states, they are dispositional in nature and may develop into character traits: "our traits are shaped by our emotions and moods, just as our emotions and moods are shaped by our traits" (Goldie, 2000: 141). Figure 8.1 roughly presents the main characteristics of moods and affects in such a way that their oppositional nature becomes clear. Examples of moods as opposed to affects are anxiety as opposed to fear, sadness (as opposed to) grief, euphoria/ joy, dysphoria/anger, tedium/boredom.

The Person between Moods and Affects

Moods and affects are oppositional extremes in the person's emotional experience and are characterized by different constellations of feelings and by different temporal, intentional, and narrative patterns.

Mood	Affect
Unfocused	Focused
Non-intentional	Intentional
Not motivated	Motivated
Inarticulate	Articulate
Horizontal absorption	No horizontal absorption
Emanated from, not by	Emanated from and by
No captivation	Captivation
No "felt causes"	"Felt causes"
Indefinite and indeterminate	Determinate
No directedness	Directedness
	Instantaneous

Adapted, with slight modifications, from the list found in Smith (1986: 109–111).

Figure 8.1 Mood and affect

Intentionality

Intentionality is the aspect of a psychic state to be "of" or "about" something. The standard phenomenological view on moods and affects is more or less clear on one fundamental difference: moods are unintentional and affects intentional. However, this view may be modified by relating the two feeling-states to the person. It is correct to say that an affect such as fear is about the particular object of fear (e.g. the bear), and that an anxious mood does not point to any specific intentional object, but manifests itself as an unarticulated background tonality or atmosphere that contaminates my whole field of awareness. Nevertheless, my mood seems to contaminate the way I relate to the world in the sense that it is accompanied by a certain atmosphere in my perceptions. A situation that beforehand would not intimidate me at all now fills me with an irresistible desire to run away and look for protection. The feelings involved in the intentional attitude of my affects are indeed changed by my current mood. My mood is expressed by how perceptions or thoughts affect me. Moods materialize in affects in that I am affected through my mood. This may suggest a covert intentionality in moods. Whereas affects have a direct and clear intentional object (an object of perception or a thought), moods are characterized by multiple objects (Siemer, 2005). Whereas affects point to an explicit experience such as a dangerous situation, a happy smile, a beautiful landscape, a difficult task, and so on, moods, on the contrary, point to my being the person I am in a given situation. Moods can be compared with what Ricoeur calls "ontological sentiments" in that "[t]hey denote the fundamental feeling ... namely, man's very openness to being" (1960: 120). We can say that whereas affects point forward towards a specific object, moods point inward towards my being the person I am. More precisely, moods contain a bipolar intentionality in the sense that they often materialize in a certain affect owing to an explicit object, but at the same time point to my being the person I am, and thereby awake questions, doubts, considerations, evaluations, and finally deliberations about my-being-this-person.

Temporality

The concept of temporality is understood in terms of how the person experiences time and how the existence of the person is inevitably formed and developed in time. Temporality is, therefore, a subjective modality of the concept of time; time is considered a constitutive part of both the being and the subjective experience of the person. The person changes through time and experiences how the world, other people, and herself change in time. Temporality is not time as an exclusively private or pure cosmological phenomenon, but both time as experienced and lived by the person and time as working on and with the person.

Moods and affects display different temporal patterns. Affects are often briefer than moods. They captivate me, occupy my whole field of awareness, and thereby move me to a determinate action within a restricted period of time. Moods, on the contrary, may last for days, weeks, or even years in that they paralyze my thoughts and retain me from acting (sadness) or throw me into weird actions without any thoughts of the past or the future (euphoria). The intensity of the feelings involved in affects demands a concrete action regarding our present situation such as to express our anger, escape the bear, return the happy smile, work on the difficult task, and so on. Obviously, we often do not act out of the affect but restrain ourselves from acting out of it. We can dominate the affect by cognition. For example, the irresistible desire to insult or thump a malicious boss may be suppressed by the fear of losing my job. The intensity of the affect then gradually subsides, and I turn my attention to other matters. This, however, does not imply that the affect vanishes altogether. It may remain as a bitter memory that brings forth unpleasant feelings every time it pops up in my mind (Goldie, 2000: 149–151).

What really matters in the therapeutic interview is the dialectic of moods and affects through time. Affects may transform themselves into moods and finally become a permanent part of our "character"; moods may determine affects because they alter the way we are affected by objects and thoughts. Last, but not least, a given mood may become an affect when in reflection I can articulate it and find its motivations and "felt causes," that is, the way it roots me in a given situation.

An affect may transform itself into a mood that imposes itself on me for days or longer (grief can transform into a general sadness; anger into dysphoria; boredom into tedium). Thus, a mood may develop out of an affect as the affect itself loses its instantaneous, focused, and motivated character. Also, a mood might not be the product of a single affect and the following action or suppression of action, but a constellation of feelings elicited in several episodes. Moods (e.g. irritability, sadness, tedium, euphoria) change the way I am affected by the world (and my own thoughts) in that they predispose my field of attention (thus my conscious experience) in a certain way. And, as we have seen, in the course of time, moods may – in virtue of being dispositional – transform themselves into an inherent and permanent part of my self. An affect can develop into a mood, and a mood can develop into a basic emotional tonality. For instance, a dysphoric state can gain such a hold on my person that it turns into a certain trait, for example an irritable, hostile, mean, polemical, misanthropic, or adverse character. This basic emotional tonality is a permanent, implicit protention, or readiness to (re)act and be affected in a given way, and probably also to develop certain moods more than others. In this way, emotions become an essential part of a person, of one's sense of personal identity. This feeling of sameness comes close to what Ricoeur (1992) calls "character." This basic emotional tonality is usually tacit and I notice it only when it is not there. It is important to notice that all these transformations from affects to moods to character occur pre-reflectively and without a deliberate and thematic involvement of the person in the process, whereas the transformation of a mood into an affect involves reflection.

A special kind of enduring emotions are *passions*. Passions are long-standing tendencies that represent an abnormal break in the otherwise ceaseless ebb and flow of our emotional life. A passion is a persistent, pervasive, and ego-synthonic emotional trait that becomes incorporated into one's identity and provides a stable normative structure through which a substantial proportion of relations with the environment are evaluated.

Narrativity

Narrativity indicates that a significant part of a person's self-experience and self-understanding is based on self-narratives – an ongoing process of establishing coherent formulations about who I am, who I was, and where I am going. Through self-narratives I seek to understand my actions and experiences as a semantically coherent pattern of chronologically ordered elements, and to grasp the way I relate myself to that understanding and to the world. We tend to constitute our experiences and our identity through self-narratives. The temporal aspect of our being becomes emphasized in the narrative approach to personhood. We are changing every second of our life, and yet we feel that we remain (almost) the same person. Our identity prevails through time, even though our body may alter and deform, and our ideas may change drastically. Although our identity prevails, we may change as persons during our life span. Thus, identity – in the sense of personal identity – is not mere sameness.

Personal identity is formed through a dialectic of two forms of identity: Being-the-Same and Being-Oneself (Ricoeur, 1992). The fundamental trait of Being-the-Same is permanence in time. The set of distinctive marks which permit the reidentification of a human individual as being the same is called "character" (Ricoeur, 1992: 119). My character is that in which my feeling of remaining the same in time and through changes is rooted, and that by which other people identify and describe me.

However, I do not coincide with my character. Being who I am involves another kind of identity: an identity constituted in Being-Oneself. Whereas my character is determined by my past actions, random events, and contingent factors that are now out of my control (Ricoeur, 1950: 343), my identity as Being-Oneself, on the contrary, depends on how I voluntarily relate myself to being a person with this particular character. Being-Oneself is constituted by my active relation to my character. This implies self-continuity and responsibility not as a contingent, but as an essential component of personhood. Both these dimensions are mainly shaped through self-narratives.

How, then, do moods and affects figure in the dialectic of Being-the-Same and Being-Oneself developed in the narrative structure of self-experience? A given mood can develop itself into a character trait, that is, a permanent part of one's sense of personal identity; this transformation occurs pre-reflexively and without a deliberate and thematic involvement of the person. Through narratives, moods can also be incorporated actively, reflectively, and thematically into a person's identity. Moods are connected to self-understanding. I understand who I am in the context of my practical engagement, as embedded in a certain world (private and social), and this engagement is primordially enveloped in a certain feeling-state. My questioning about myself is often elicited by my mood (and by disturbing affects that disclose my mood) before my identity becomes an explicit problem. Moods may disclose to me what word and deeds do not. Feeling-states are no hindrance to "cognitive" knowledge. The possibility of self-disclosure, which belongs to moods and affects, is fundamental for cognition in that a given mood can point to a breach in the way I, reflectively, understand myself. I can be locked up in my own way of thinking, chained to my thoughts in such a way that my formulations about myself reflect a wrong or at least problematic understanding of my personhood. Although our capability to choose to be what (who) we want to be is a constitutive feature of personhood, these choices (evaluations) are always tied to the involuntary aspect of my personhood (Grøn, 2004).

To summarize: although emotions are universal among most living creatures, the human experience of emotions is drastically different from that of other animals since a human person is a contextualized self with intentional attitudes capable of position-taking, i.e. evaluation and deliberation.

The feeling that an emotion elicits is an essential component of the emotion itself and we, as persons, need to acknowledge this feeling to fully access the emotion. To differentiate among different emotional experiences we need to pay attention to the diffuse and vague constellation of feelings involved in our interaction with the world.

Feelings make a fundamental contribution to uncover a person's situatedness in the world. We as persons can understand ourselves and the world in which we are situated through the awareness of our practical engagement, and this engagement is primordially enveloped in a certain feeling-state.

Emotions may display different phenomenal patterns. Therefore, we need different concepts for moods and affects. Moods are unfocused, non-intentional, not motivated, and unarticulated, whereas affects are intentional, motivated, and articulated.

Emotions are fundamental in the process of narrative identity since they may disclose problems in the stories we formulate about ourselves. They disclose the fact that our formulations can be right or wrong and elicit the need for modifying the story we tell about ourselves.

Chapter

9 What Are Values and Why Are They Relevant to the Therapeutic Interview?

"Values" is one of those terms that although familiar in everyday discourse has no settled meaning. Values are "what matters" or "is important." But what matters or is important covers a wide range of concepts (needs, desires, preferences, virtues, etc.), the meanings of which are both individually complex (reflecting as they do the variety of personal, cultural, and historical values) and collectively conflicting (what we desire and what we value as virtuous are often in conflict for example).

Values are attitudes that regulate the felt-meanings of the world and the significant actions of the person, being organized into concepts that do not arise from rational activity but rather within the sphere of feelings. Thus, grasping the values of a person is key to understanding her way of understanding and representing herself and the surrounding world. In general, comprehending a person's values is a key to understanding her "form of life" or "being in the world," that is, the "pragmatic motive" and the "system of relevance" that determine the meaning structure of the world she lives in, and regulate her style of experience and action (Stanghellini, 2016a).

Although what is valued is framed cognitively (it is thought, perceived, remembered, imagined, etc.), actually attaching value (valuing something as good, or bad, or with indifference) always involves emotions. Values are beliefs, but not cold beliefs. Valuing is a process rooted in the emotional dimension of life. Comparative emotions are essential to the conative processes of deciding and choosing. Valuing entails comparative emotions since it is through comparing emotions that we value something as better or worse than something else. Ethics as a whole, and the value system of a given person, is, first and foremost, a matter of emotional experience, not a matter of general principles justifying pre-set rules of right conduct (Husserl, 1988). Thus an account of value experience comprises cognitive as well as affective and conative elements.

Values are also interwoven with personal identity. Scheler (1927/1973), along with most other phenomenologists, took the emotional faculty to be essential for moral values. Persons experience themselves simultaneously at different levels, caught "in between" the possibilities of good and evil, of spirit and flesh, of God and animal life. The complex and conflicting nature of value experience becomes clear in the richly detailed account Scheler (1928/2012) gives of shame and repentance. First, as to the complexity of value experience, in Scheler's account it emerges as a consequence of the tension between the animal and the divine by which the human condition is uniquely characterized. This means that our values are necessarily *stratified*: there are values of the Holy and Unholy (the Divine), psychic values (the Beautiful and the Ugly, Right and Wrong, Truth and Falsehood), vital values (Noble and Vulgar), sensual values (the Agreeable and the Disagreeable), and values of utility (Economics, Government) (Figure 9.1).

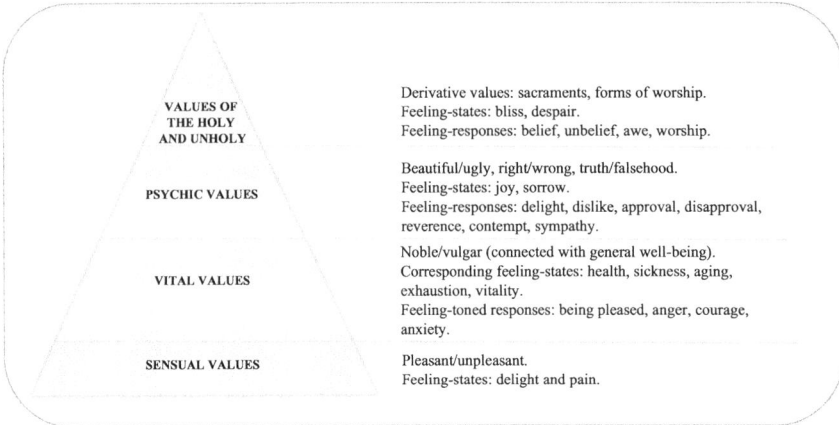

Figure 9.1 Scheler's hierarchy of values

Second, as to the conflicting nature of values, this is a necessary rather than merely contingent feature of the human condition. The basic condition for feeling shame is an imbalance between the claims of spiritual personhood and embodied needs. In shame what Scheler characterizes as "spirit" and "flesh," eternity and time, essence and existence, come together in tension. To be a human person is to experience simultaneously these two orders of being such that one is unable to sever either without losing one's very humanity.

Yet it is in this tension too that the possibility of repentance arises. To be a person means to be able to acknowledge and consequently extinguish in repenting one's having-been-bad while simultaneously becoming good. Scheler's account of repentance thus highlights, in a way that goes beyond the resources of merely cognitive strategies to deal with values, the dynamic and temporal nature of personhood and of personal values.

Two essential dimensions of value experience are balanced decisions and mutual respect. Ricoeur's value theory (1950) involves three basic concepts: motivation, feelings, and imagination. Values are based on motivations, ranging from bodily motivations to motivations of pure reason. Bodily motivations are involuntary and bound to our basic needs such as thirst and hunger. Rational motivations are voluntary and include the capacity to transcend our bodily needs.

Like Scheler then, Ricoeur shows, in this case through his concept of motivations, how values come into conflict one with another. Ricoeur goes further, however, in giving us an account of how we resolve value conflicts through the exercise of feelings and imagination. Feelings, understood as spontaneous beliefs about what is good or bad, highlight motives and it is the relative strengths of our feelings that produce actions. For instance, I decide not to follow the bodily motive of hunger where this is outweighed by the rational motive of keeping in shape. Imagination is what enables a person to break with the immediate satisfaction of a bodily motive. It is through imaginative comparison that we are able to compare one motive with another and to balance their respective satisfactions.

Each person feels a given value in a given state of affairs. This value is pre-reflectively felt rather than reflectively established. Or better: it is sensed before it can be cognitively acknowledged. Also, each person has her hierarchy of values which reflects her hierarchy of involuntary motivations. Thus Scheler's and Ricoeur's exploration of the hierarchical nature of values gives us a rich account of the process of balanced decisions.

It is the hierarchy of values one establishes by acting in a given way that constitutes one's personal identity. Yet this identity is necessarily unstable since we live in a social world and encounter other persons with their own often very different hierarchies. This leads to a quest for legitimacy, for the recognition of our values by others. But the quest is mutual. Our own values, therefore, to the extent that they embody our identity as unique individuals, are rooted in and depend critically on the mutuality of human relationships.

The constitution of the person as a healthy individual can only be realized within an intersubjective framework: the Other is needed to achieve basic trust, respect, and integrity. These realizations can only be achieved through the experience of the Other's *recognition*. Self-recognition, that is, the recognition of oneself as capable of certain realizations, requires at any step the recognition of the Other (Ricoeur, 2004).

The need and the desire to be recognized as an individual person, and as part of a human society, to be accepted, respected, forgiven, and loved is a fundamental value in human existence – as well as eating and staying alive. My existence is conditioned and articulated by the value of social recognition alongside the organic values of my biological life. Yet the need for recognition can even be stronger than other needs rooted in my organic values. The passion to achieve recognition may go beyond the animal struggle for self-preservation or domination. Recognition is not a struggle for life, rather a struggle to tear from the other an avowal, an attestation, a proof of my value as a person. Sometimes this struggle for recognition is a struggle against life (Ricoeur, 2004). We as human persons can choose to renounce, at least in part, our material gains (e.g. a part of one's salary) in order to achieve social recognition (e.g. respect, dignity, and the acknowledgment of one's capacities) (Honneth, 2008).

The analyses of recognition, from a sociological and political standpoint, show that the experience of recognition is indispensable to achieve basic trust, a sense of autonomy, the confidence that is necessary to articulate one's needs and desires, and to put into use one's own skills and capacities.

There are three paradigmatic forms of recognition (Honneth, 2008). The first is *Love*, whereby the person experiences the recognition of his particular needful nature in order to attain that affective security that allows him to articulate his needs. The prototype of this is the experience of parental care. This form of recognition is necessary to achieve "basic trust," that is, to trust oneself. The second is *Law*: the subject experiences that juridical institutions guarantee the recognition of his autonomy. This form of recognition is necessary to achieve "respect," that is, to respect oneself. The third is *Solidarity*: the subject experiences the recognition of the value of his own capacities. This form of recognition is necessary to achieve "integrity," that is, to feel a meaningful part of society and to contribute with one's capacities to sustain other subjects and, reciprocally, to be sustained by them. These three forms of recognition are basic requirements for the good life. They cannot be achieved by the subject as an individual separated from the others. They can be achieved only through *interaction*, that is, through the *experience* of recognition.

Valuing the value of recognition is the starting point for developing an idea of care based on value-acknowledgment and value-pluralism. Persons have reasons to live differently. And our patients' values depart from common-sense values as they are embedded in life-worlds that are different from each other and from our own. There is an axiological dimension in mental disorders. This axiological dimension is a component of human suffering that descriptive psychopathology (and even more so, clinical psychiatry) has often disregarded (Sadler, 2005). The neglect of the value system of persons suffering from mental disorders contributes to seeing them merely as people who bear pathological experiences and beliefs; this may have a stigmatizing effect on them and contribute to judging some of these people's actions as meaningless and incomprehensible.

Value-recognition reflects the ideal of *modus vivendi* (Gray, 2010), whose aim is not looking for consensus about the best values, or sharing common values in order to live together in peace. Rather, it aims to find terms in which different forms of life can coexist.

Modus vivendi is a kind of practice whose aim is not to still the conflict of value. It is to reconcile individuals and ways of life honoring conflicting values. "We do not need common values in order to live together in peace. We need institutions in which many forms of life can coexist" (Gray, 2010: 25).

Our inherited ideal of toleration accepts with regret the fact that there are many ways of life. The good is plural. There is no one good that is right. And there is no one solution between conflicting goods that is right. "It is not that there can be no right solution in such conflicts. Rather, there are many" (Gray, 2010: 26). The idea of dialogue as a means to universal consensus should be given up. The project of *modus vivendi* among ways of life animated by permanently diverging values should take its place.

The practice that derives from this supports the patient in the search for value-acknowledgment, that is, insight, understanding, resilience, and development of self-management abilities, rather than merely focusing on symptom assessment and reduction (Fulford, 1999). Also, this practice enhances value-pluralism, that is, an idea of care that aims at a relation of coexistence rather than consensus.

Most of our current, supposedly "humanitarian" or "dialogic" therapeutic practices are based on the ideal of establishing some form of consensus between patients and carers, or between patients and the social milieu. Yet, consensus is a woolly kind of "dialogic" value. While it looks for agreement and harmony, it implicitly holds that some values are better than others and builds on the metaphysical belief that conflict of values is just a stage on the way to sharing universal values. In this vein, conflicts of values are signs of imperfection, rather a constitutive part of human life. This unrealistic idea promotes pseudo-dialogic practices that downplay the person's subjectivity and surreptitiously endorse one-sided values. Examples of this are "social rehabilitation" (which endorses prevailing social values), or potentially intolerant techniques to enhance "compliance" (which endorse the distinction illness/health based on the clinician's values) – both taking for granted that "good" values are on the side of the clinician.

Coexistence with mental sufferers and with the values each of them embodies is better practice. This practice is produced in dialogue, which is contact across a distance. It aims to acknowledge, understand, and respect different ways of life, enlighten our ethical conflicts, honor conflicting values – and finally negotiate reciprocal recognition.

The Therapeutic Interview as a Quest for Meaning

10

The therapeutic interview is a quest for meaning. A tentative framework for the therapeutic interview includes five levels of meaningfulness. We will illustrate this, following the case study of Giacomo explored in Chapter 8, in which the myth of nature as a harmonious order is reversed with the resultant vision of the garden as a place of *universal suffering*. The garden, viewed by common sense as a place of beauty, vitality, and growth, is seen by Giacomo as pure chaos – as a blind and mechanistic world of decay and destruction, evil and monstrosity.

As we have seen, there is an analogy between Giacomo's vision of the garden and the life-world of people affected by contamination obsession. In both cases, the central themes are death and decay. The patients affected by contamination obsession are "dominated by horror and dread," Straus (1948: 10) writes, "not because of fear of death which may hit them in the near future, but because of the presence of death in sensory immediateness, warded off in disgust." To Giacomo, these feelings and thoughts are totally egosyntonic.

As shown in Chapter 5, in the course of the therapeutic interview we approach the symptom – as well as any other phenomena – as a *text*. The "reader" is in the position of understanding a text better than the author himself – and the author can understand himself better by reflecting on the text he has produced, by unfolding, in the text, the world which it conveys. The text, as with Heraclitus's understanding of the Oracle's dicta, neither says nor hides – it *discloses*. Five levels of meaningfulness can be made visible through the therapeutic interview: unfolding; the emotional core; narrative appropriation; personal values; and importance.

Unfolding

The first step of the therapeutic interview is the unfolding of the phenomenal world the patients live in – the world as it is felt and seen from their first-person perspective, the phenomenal world, the world as it appears to the subject of experience, including all those details that resist standard semiological classification. Unfolding means to explicate, expound, exposit, expand, open out, open up, unfurl, spread out, lay bare the pleats, folds, doubles, plications, flexions, flexures, creases, corrugations, wrinkles of a text. The opposite of this is to garble, pervert, distort, twist/stretch/strain the text itself.

What comes into sight is the texture of the world that is immanent in the text itself, although it may remain unknown to or unnoticed by the author. Now we can see that the aim of this process is to rescue the sense or internal coherence among the clinical (as well as existential) phenomena entailed in a given condition of suffering. The first level of meaningfulness of a text is the way a text belongs to itself. The guidelines for this kind of analysis, as we have seen in Chapter 6, are so called *existentialia*, that is, the basic structures of subjectivity within which each single experience is situated, and include lived time, space, body, and otherness.

The unfolding consists in bringing out (i) the raw feelings of the patient's experiences and (ii) the personal sense that the patient attributes to his experiences (Stanghellini, 2007). At this level of the analysis of Giacomo's world we find the physiognomy of decay.

As we have seen, disorder, decay, decomposition, and death are not just themes in Giacomo's world-view or "philosophy of life." Rather, they are *felt* like real entities in his life-world whose presence haunts the space near him. In the following, we will call Giacomo's life-world *the garden of universal souffrance*. Giacomo feels the world along with the physiognomy of decay – the loss of the natural and habitual forms of things in the world. Microbes, coming from the putrescent surrounding world, can rapidly invade and infect space.

Of special relevance for the appearing of the garden of universal souffrance is a metamorphosis of lived distance as the key feature of the spatial structure – the relation between the person and things in space. Giacomo experiences a lack of distance from anything and feels surrounded and besieged. This extreme proximity to things is accompanied by a metamorphosis of materiality – the way things appear to the person. The excessive nearness of things to the person makes him feel on the surface of things – as if he could see things through a microscope – what would normally be invisible: contamination substances like microbes. Contamination can be so rapid because distance between things is so small. Microbes can rapidly invade such a space because there is no distance to cover.

Acceleration is the key character of lived time in the garden of universal souffrance. Things are not felt as stable; instead they conceal rapid biological processes that cause decay. Time inexorably vanishes and inexorably passes away. The dripping of water, the ticking of the clock are intolerable because they remind the person that life passes away. Life may be dominated by the paralyzing threat of approaching death. While *tempus fugit*, existence has come to a standstill.

As a consequence of this, Giacomo's behavior may be characterized by extreme orderliness and perfectionism. He may spend most of his time in extenuating rituals aimed at eliminating disorder and dirt. Sometimes he is prey to terror and feels he is surrounded by a terrifying power and tries to defend himself from the aggression of a threatening world by confining himself to a more and more restricted space.

The Emotional Core

The *second stratum* of meaningfulness made visible by the therapeutic process is the invisible condition of possibility of the visible world that appears in the first level.

This is the structural level strictly speaking: looking for the structure that transpires through each phenomenon of the world and keeps these phenomena meaningfully interconnected. Also, the way the text belongs to the type of (embodied) consciousness in which it takes place, or the way the text belongs to the being-in-the-world displayed by the text. This is an exploration in the structure of consciousness. It looks for the way consciousness must be structured to make phenomena appear as they appear to the experiencing person.

A given life-world is not simply a casual association of (normal or abnormal) phenomena. The manifold phenomena are meaningfully interconnected, i.e. they form a structure. Now, to have a phenomenological grasp on these phenomena is to grasp the structural nexus that lend coherence and continuity to them, since each phenomenon in a structure carries the traces of the underlying form of subjectivity. Looking for structural relationships consists in the unfolding of the basic structure(s) of subjectivity, i.e. the way the person appropriates phenomena.

At this level of analysis we find an *emotion*. As shown in detail in Chapter 8, emotions are kinetic, dynamic forces that drive us in our ongoing interactions with the environment. Emotions are protentional states in the sense that they project the person into the future providing a felt readiness for action (Gallagher, 2005). Feelings make up a crucial part of emotions. Feelings are the primordial medium in which I encounter the world as a set of affordances: a set of relevant possibilities that are my own possibilities as a person situated in this particular world. We feel and perceive the world in a certain way because of our being-in-the-world. The significance of an event or state of affairs is not merely a matter of its intrinsic properties, but rather of its relation to me and my current engagement. Feelings reveal how the world is for me. We can only understand ourselves and the world in which we are situated through the context of our practical engagement, and, as we have seen, this engagement is primordially enveloped in a certain feeling-state.

Disgust is the basic emotion accompanying the garden of universal souffrance experience. It is a kind of nausea accompanying the perception of decay. Disgust as an emotion displays the basic attitude that persons like Giacomo[1] have in relation to their world. As such, the emotion of disgust can disclose the deep metamorphosis the life-world has undergone. Disgust is linked by the perception of decay – what Straus calls *aneidos*, i.e. the loss of form of a given thing in the world. Disgust occurs when things lose their integrity, as in the case of putrefaction, or when a part is separated from its whole. In the garden of universal souffrance experience most of the world is perceived along with the physiognomy of decay. For Giacomo the world is not inhabited by living things that appear as opportunities in the process of life, but by mere matter destined to decompose and die. The world Giacomo lives in has such a structure that he feels the presence of death in sensory immediateness and the near future. The very same atmosphere is conveyed by W. B. Yeats's poem "Sailing to Bizantium":

> That is no country for old men. The young
>   In one another's arms, birds in the trees
> – Those dying generations – at their song,
> The salmon-falls, the mackerel-crowded seas,
> Fish, flesh, or fowl, commend all summer long
>   Whatever is begotten, born, and dies.

The "crowd" of beings depicted in these lines, rather than suggesting the idea of life and the atmosphere of vitality, insinuate a feeling of decay and the phobic-disgust atmosphere with its characteristic lack of distance between each entity in space that makes them appear as menacing; and the acceleration of time that makes things appear as unstable and decaying. We can trace this transformation of the life-world back to a metamorphosis of embodied consciousness. Thus an analysis of disgust as the basic emotion characterizing the garden of universal souffrance reveals the very source of the spatiotemporal architecture of this world.

---

[1] In the case of Giacomo Leopardi, disgust may be moderated by a philosophical stance, as the quest for objectivity, or for "right and pity," as is the case for his last poem *La ginestra* ("Broom, or the flower of desert," 2002).

This kind of life-world arises from the phobic *disgust atmosphere* (von Gebsattel, 1954). This is a "disintegration phenomenon" (Bürgy, 2007): in the disgust atmosphere, the integration of parts of one's experiences into the whole structure of consciousness is missing. Therefore, entities in this universe appear like alien elements for the experiencing person, like islands in the stream of her mental course (von Gebsattel, 1954). Disgust as well as the physiognomy of decay belong to the person's conscious experience, but the way disgust brings about the metamorphosis from a well-integrated world into a disintegrated one, i.e. the relationship between the emotion of disgust and the physiognomy of decay, may remain unconscious.

Narrative Appropriation

The *third level* of meaningfulness made manifest by this exploration is the world that the text opens up in the patient when it is appropriated by the clinician. The clinician "appropriates" the sense of the patient's experience and suggests his view over it. To appropriate the patient's text means to acknowledge the way the text belongs to the clinician, to his ownmost possibilities, the way the clinician could inhabit it.

In doing so, he makes explicit his understanding as his own, i.e. the vantage point from which he sees the situation. Through this process a liminal, dual mode of understanding is established, revealing differences as well as points of intersection (Stanghellini and Lysaker, 2007). At this level, we can situate the construct called by Straus *aneidos*. This is a metaphor, a product of imagination or illustration meant to represent the *loss of good form* of the world the person with contamination obsession lives in, and make sense of his behaviors. The clinician may reason like this: "If it ever happened to me to live in a world abandoned by all form, order, or structure (*Gestalt*), then I would behave exactly as Giacomo, restricting my space to a tiny but safe corner, and defending myself against ruinous time speed by performing magic rituals of control." Or: "In order to make sense of Giacomo's otherwise absurd and meaningless narratives and behavior, I must imagine him as living in a world that has completely lost its *eidos* or form."

All understanding is an attempt at reducing the distance between the text and its reader. A first level of meaningfulness, as we have seen, emerges from a structure as its internal organization via a process of unfolding based on a linguistic exchange. The further level of meaningfulness at issue here emerges as the negotiation between the subjectivity of the patient and that of the clinician. We may call the first "sense" and the second "meaning."

How does this happen in practice? It happens through the negotiation of narratives. As patterns of meanings that emerge during this process, narratives contribute to create points of contact between two subjectivities (Atwood and Stolorow, 1984) – namely: *inter-views* (Figure 10.1). There is a requirement of exchange between the interviewer's narrative about the interviewee's experiences and the way the latter makes sense of them. The upshot of this exchange is connecting the horizon of sense of the patient with that of the clinician. The benchmark of this process of intersubjective understanding is *not* a shared narrative, rather the capacity of this process to enhance each person's acknowledgment of the point of view of the Other, and by doing so improve one's capacity to sense one's experiences as one's own and reflect upon them taking an intentional stance over them (Stanghellini, 2007). The capacity of acknowledging the point of view of the Other, and enhancing a capacity for reflection, are also the basic goals of the process of the therapeutic interview.

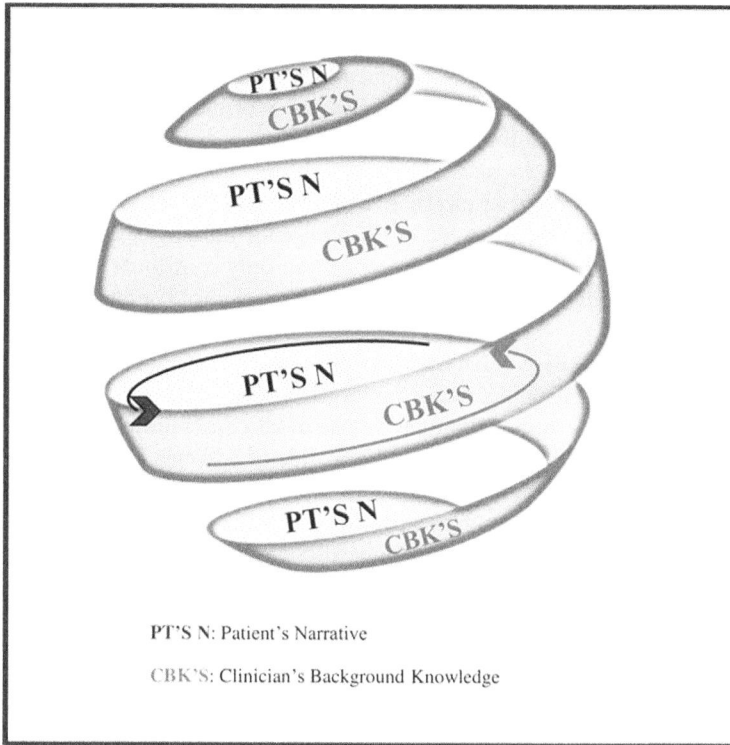

PT'S N: Patient's Narrative

CBK'S: Clinician's Background Knowledge

Figure 10.1 Patient's/clinician's inter-views

In the case of my dialogue with Giacomo, I would say that I don't see the garden as he sees it, but I could see it as the icon of universal souffrance if I were taken by a feeling of disgust, or if I were committed to an uncompromising and implacable stance of objectivity. I would then encourage Giacomo to unfold his feelings (e.g. disgust) and his values (e.g. objectivity and awareness as the greatest goods) as the pragmatic motives for his style of experience and action.

Personal Values

Values are the *fourth* level of meaningfulness. As shown in Chapter 9, values are attitudes that regulate meaning-bestowing and the significant actions of the person, being organized into concepts that do not arise from rational activity but rather within the sphere of feelings. Unfolding Giacomo's values helps in grasping the "pragmatic motive" and the "system of relevance" that determine the meaning structure of the world he lives in, and regulate his style of experience and action.

If we ask Giacomo to spell out his values we will soon realize that they are coherently organized in a specific world-view. Obviously, this is not the case with all persons having a world-view. The majority may have a more or less confused practical philosophy, so to say, without a sound empirical basis and logically inconsistent. Giacomo has a lucid and consistent philosophy of life. The basic value of Giacomo's attitude or mental framework is *objectivity*. Objectivity is to him the attitude to establish a rational world picture in the face of a mythological and faith-driven *fabula* about the world. An objective attitude also praises clarity in the face of obscurity.

The only valuable knowledge, he holds, is that obtained through the cruel analysis of the real. This crude realism inescapably brings one to the awareness of the "triple *nulla*": we *know* nothing, we *are* nothing, there is nothing *after* death. The real is exactly what one can see in the garden of universal souffrance: chaos increases with our desire for pleasure and happiness, the unhappiest moment is that of pleasure.

Awareness and self-awareness are the outcome of this praise for objectivity and rationality. Yet, Giacomo is also aware that greater self-awareness can only contribute to greater unhappiness. Also, he knows that his objective attitude, fed by unprejudiced perception, can ossify and become lifeless.

He would ironically conclude: "Life is tragic, yet let's not make a tragedy out of it!" He rejects all escapes from his tragic sense of life, including forgetfulness – the regression to the dullness of matter itself – and distraction – the total eclipse of all consciousness. Incidentally, these are the values at work respectively in the life-worlds of addicted and of manic persons.

To be noted, Giacomo's values should not be mistaken for some kind of delusion, or wrong beliefs, and thus treated with some sort of orthopaedics of abnormal cognition. It is of capital importance to rescue values from the jungle of symptoms. Acknowledging the other person's values is a source of understanding and reciprocal recognition.

Recognition is a task, a kind of emotional and intellectual readiness to acknowledge the reasons of the other person. This task culminates in acknowledging the values inherent to the other person's world-view. Recognizing the other person is to acknowledge the existential difference, the particular autonomy, which separates me from the way of being in the world that characterizes him. Any forgetting of this difference will be an obstacle to recognition since the other may live in a life-world whose structure is (at least in part) different from my own. I need to set aside my own pre-reflexive, natural attitude, and to approach the other's world as I would do while exploring an unknown and alien country. I need to be interested in the invisible semantic ordering of the world the other person lives in. I also must acknowledge that it belongs to my ownmost possibilities as a vulnerable human being. Finally, I need to concede that the way of being in the world of that individual person transcends the concrete situation of that person herself and can thus be envisioned as a universal phenomenon since it belongs to human existence as such.

Importance

The *fifth* level is the existence of that being in the world as a universal problem. The way the text belongs to human existence, to the *condició humana*.

In the process of unfolding and interpretation described above, the meanings that we find in the text may exceed or transcend the concrete situation of their production and be re-enacted in new contexts – universal contexts. The text may display meanings that transcend the situation in which the text was produced and may reveal themselves as a priori conditions of human existence. "To understand an author better than he can understand himself is to unfold the revelatory power implicit in his discourse, beyond the limited horizon of his own existential situation" (Ricoeur, 1981: 191). Ricoeur calls this the *importance* of a text. The importance of a text is what "goes 'beyond' its relevance to the initial situation" (Ricoeur, 1981: 207). It displays meanings that exceed or transcend the concrete situation of their production and may be re-enacted in new contexts. In virtue of its importance a text acquires a universal (not merely contingent) meaning, and the author personifies a universal problem (he stops being merely a contingent sufferer). This is the supreme instantiation of the phenomenological-hermeneutic unconscious.

Giacomo's attitude towards the garden is driven by a theoretical reflexive interest rather than a practical pre-reflexive one. He is more interested in seeing in the garden a piece of evidence confirming his tragic world-view than in getting involved in the garden in terms of more earthly needs and desires. We could also say that his interest is driven by spiritual rather than organic values – his interest is, so to say, *disembodied*.

As far as the garden of universal souffrance (and contamination obsession) is concerned, its importance consists in revealing the role of embodied consciousness in organizing our world of senses. The order of the world is not given a priori, rather it is the effect or projection of an implicit *enactment* or act of consciousness that imposes an order on it. *Giacomo has a disembodied interest in the garden.* The outcome of the absence, or disruption –whatever its cause could be – of the implicit and automatic link between Giacomo's body and the garden decrees the "catastrophe of the world" (De Martino, 2002) as we normally experience it in our common-sense cognition. This catastrophe of the familiarity of the world paves the way to an alternative experience of the world that in our case study is rigidly organized around the value of objectivity and the core emotion of disgust. Giacomo's *objective* attitude, driven by disembodied perception, discloses the vision of death in the place where common-sense embodied perception would see life. The fifth level of meaningfulness of Giacomo's case study is that all sorts of objectivity are indeed the consequence of a given enactment or attitude towards the world. Giacomo's "objectivity" is thus not "objective" in the sense that it reflects the ultimate essence of reality; rather, it is an "objectification" of his subjective values and emotion-driven attitude.

Chapter 11

Guidelines for the Therapeutic Interview
The PHD Method

In the previous chapter, we explained the basic principles of the therapeutic interview as a quest for meaning. In this chapter we will provide the practical guidelines for performing the therapeutic interview according to these principles. The practice of care that derives from them is based on the integration of three basic dispositives, synthesized in the acronym PHD: Phenomenology, Hermeneutics, Psycho-Dynamics (Stanghellini, 2016a, 2016b).

Phenomenological Unfolding (P)

The basic purpose of the unfolding is to empower both clinician and patient with a systematic knowledge of the abnormal phenomena that affect the patient. "Unfolding" means to open up and lay bare the pleats of the patient's experiences. We already illustrated the meaning and purpose of unfolding in the previous chapter through the example of Giacomo's garden of universal souffrance and the atmosphere of decay that permeates it. What comes into sight is the texture that is immanent in the patient's style of experience/ action, although it may remain invisible to or unnoticed by him. Unfolding enriches understanding by providing further resources in addition to those which are immediately visible. In the case of the garden of universal souffrance, Giacomo's life-world is dominated by the paralyzing threat of approaching death and as a defense from this he spends most of his time in extenuating rituals aimed at reducing decay. The main aim of unfolding is to rescue the *logos* of the phenomena in themselves, that is, immanent in the intertwining of phenomena – in our case study we called this (after Straus) the *aneidos* or the loss of form, order, and structure of the world.

An outstanding example of phenomenological unfolding is given by Minkowski (1930/ 1993; see detailed discussion in Stanghellini, 2010). In a classic idiographic essay on the structure of depressive states, following an in-depth portrayal of the manifold abnormal experiences and sensations of a 26-year-old man with a diagnosis of "ambivalent depres- sion" (a subtype of major depression), mainly relying on this man's self-descriptions, Minkowski attempts to grasp the kernel underlying these symptoms. The patient reports his complaints and Minkowski carefully registers and systematically orders them. He documents cenesthopathic troubles ("I have the sensation of a stop of vegetative func- tions"), sensations of materialization ("I am nothing but a kind of animal function"), and disorders of self-awareness ("I don't feel myself anymore. I don't exist anymore") and of intersubjectivity ("I resonate with people, I reflect their vibrations," "I have the impression of being rubbish thrown into life, so much I feel distant from the others"); he complains about disorders of action ("I have always the sensation of incompleteness") and of tempor- alization ("I have been persuaded to be a person sick of time [*malade du temps*]," "I have the sensation that time passes very fast, faster than for the others, too fast and this is atrocious," "I don't have the sensation of continuity anymore," "I have the obsession of the past").

So far, Minkowski's analysis is a scholarly example of descriptive psychopathology: he records personal experiences, as idiosyncratic as they are, including those phenomena that are not categorized in ad hoc diagnostic checklists. To note, he is not simply interested in psychopathological symptoms in a traditional sense (indexes for diagnosis): he mentions neither disorders of ideation (delusions or other "false ideas") nor abnormal moods (sadness, anger, or anhedonia). Minkowski is concerned with reconstructing the patient's life-world, "the lived experience of the real world that surrounds him" (Lanteri-Laura, 1993: 108), more than counting his symptoms. To obtain this, he methodically brackets or suspends all the "ideo-affective" (cognitive and affective) contents of experience, and focuses on formal aspects or the spatiotemporal configurations that are implicit in the patient's experiences. The main guidelines for this are lived space and time, but the way the patient experiences his own body, self, and other persons are also included in Minkowski's inquiries. This patient's experiences, examined from this angle, manifest profound anomalies as compared to the common-sense world we all live in. Following this path, to a certain extent it is possible to feel or imagine what it is like to live in that world. However, at this stage of reconstruction the lived world still lacks a core that keeps its parts meaningfully interconnected – the "underlying unity characteristic of particular types of abnormal lived world" (Sass, 2001: 255).

A psychopathological syndrome is not simply an association of symptoms, but the expression of a profound and characteristic modification of the human existence in its entirety. We need to grasp the intimate transformation of subjectivity underlying the manifold symptoms and conferring on them their structural unity. In Minkowski's own words (1930/1993: 2), "the way in which personality is situated, in normal as well as in pathological terms, in relation to lived time and lived space," the "organized living unity" of abnormal psychic phenomena – a *deeper symptom* compared to surface symptoms on which contemporary nosography is based (Kendler, 2008).

The procedure here credited to Minkowski can serve as a model to grasp the *eidos* or "kernel underlying the manifest symptoms in all their variety that keeps them meaningfully interconnected or united" (Urfer, 2001: 281). To achieve the *eidos* of a given set of phenomena (in this case, the manifold of symptoms of Minkowski's patient) one can adopt a method called by phenomenology *free fantasy variation* – a series of arbitrary variations although restricted to imagined instances of the phenomenon at issue. Indeed, all the symptoms presented by Minkowski's patient can be seen as empirical variations of an essential property shared by all these symptoms. This eidetic property is the characteristic without which this set of symptoms would lose their identity (see Husserl, 1977).

In the case study illustrated by Minkowski it is the patient himself that finds the right words to talk about the *eidos* of his sufferings: *"I am a person sick of time."* This seems to be the fundamental essential phenomenon that is always implicit and virtually present in all the manifest parts of his life-world (e.g. the sensation of a stop of vegetative functions, the impression of being rubbish thrown into life, the sensation of incompleteness, the feeling that time passes very fast, the impression of a lack of continuity, and the obsession of the past).

The essential phenomenon is a disorder of the experience of time that gives the manifold of abnormal phenomena affecting this patient its meaningful coherence (more about this in Section 2). Minkowski writes that at the roots of our awareness of time there are two elements, distinct but intimately related: one dynamic in nature, preparing our *élan* towards the future, the other more static that can be called "the eternal" (*l'éternel*) (Minkowski, 1930/1993). Our normal experience of time results from their harmonious synthesis, so that time is experienced neither as a fugue nor as fixation. In pathological conditions, this synthesis falls apart. In major depressions, *élan* is overpowered by *l'éternel*. The core symptom is a disorder of conation or inhibition of becoming. This disorder of lived time transpires in all phenomena characterizing major depression, including the experience of a stagnation of endogenous vital processes, the experience of present and future dominated by the past, and the experience of the slackening of the flow of time (Stanghellini, Ballerini, et al., 2016). All are supposedly the phenomenal manifestations of the pre-phenomenal disturbance of temporality called *conation*, that is, the basic energetic momentum (*élan*) of mental life that gives the sense of aliveness and spontaneity and orientates one's life in the direction of the future. The disturbance of conation (time-sickness, *maladie du temps*) is the structural nexus that gives them unity and coherence; it allows for making sense of actions, thoughts, emotions, and experiences that would otherwise be inexplicable.

The unfolding thus helps to recover the implicit (not necessarily rejected), automatic (not censored), forgotten (not forbidden) sources that make phenomena appear as they appear to the patient, his drives, emotions, and habitus – the three emblematic components of the obscure and dissociated spontaneity that make up the involuntary dimension in human existence (Stanghellini, 2016a).

Hermeneutic Analysis (H)

The second moment of the PHD method is the analysis of the person's position-taking towards her experiences. This is called the hermeneutic moment (H) since it is focused on the way the patient interprets or makes sense of her experiences. The central idea is that there is an active interplay between the person and her basic abnormal experiences. As self-interpreting animals, we continuously strive to make sense of what happens to us, or to make a *logos* out of *pathos*. The H moment of the PHD pays attention to the active role that the person has in taking a position and interacting with her abnormal and distressing experiences. The patient, with her unique strengths and resources as well as needs and difficulties, has an active role in shaping her symptoms, and the course and outcome of her disorder.

As the P moment unfolds the patient's life-world or world-experience, the H moment reveals the patients *world-view*. This concept refers to the person's philosophy of life, i.e. the structure of values that orients her way of experiencing reality and her actions. Jaspers (1925) explains that a world-view consists of two parts: an "attitude," the pattern of mental existence by means of which the world is experienced, and a "world-picture," the whole of the mental content a person possesses. Husserl further explains that a "world-view is thus essentially an individual accomplishment, a sort of personal religious faith; but it is distinguished from traditional faith, that of revealed religion, through the fact that it makes no claim to an unconditioned truth binding for all men" (Husserl, 1936/1970: 389). A world-view is thus a mental framework or a *shelter* (*Gehause*) in which a person has her place and seeks refuge from her dread of limit situations, those situations in which her existence can be put in jeopardy (Jaspers, 1925).

Persons vulnerable to schizophrenia, for instance, may show an attitude of distrust towards conventional knowledge and attunement (Stanghellini and Ballerini, 2007).

Eccentric values in persons with schizophrenia are one aspect of an overall crisis of common sense and of these persons' difficulties in feeling attuned to others and making sense of their behavior. The outcome of this has been designated as antagonomia (literally: striving against rules) and idionomia (the sentiment of the radical uniqueness and exceptionality of one's own internal law (*nomos*) with respect to common sense or other human beings) (for details see Section 2). These quasi-philosophies are shelters or defensive housings (Jaspers, 1925). In general, we enter into one of these shelters when commonsensical assumptions are jeopardized. When I enter into one of these protective casings, it becomes a structured and structuring organization for me. My world-view protects me from the moral pain produced by disturbing experiences – as is the case with Giacomo's experience of the garden of universal souffrance – but endlessly produces other experiences of a similar kind.

In our case study, what comes into sight is Giacomo's tragic sense of life. As discussed in the previous chapter, Giacomo's values are coherently organized in a specific world-view whose kernel is *dispassionate and rational objectivity*. What is most valuable to him is to achieve an unbiased picture of the world. His praise of objectivity inescapably brings him to a form of crude realism. Giacomo is aware that his passion for objective awareness and self-awareness can only contribute to greater unhappiness. This is, at least from our point of view, an aberrant and even perverted outcome of the search for a trustworthy image of the world since we, first and foremost, strive to obtain reliable knowledge and unprejudiced perception in order to optimize our conduct, avoiding negativity (e.g. dangers) and increasing positivity (e.g. pleasure), rather than to annihilate our capacity to enjoy life. Giacomo's value of objectivity and unprejudiced perception can fossilize his life and paradoxically bias his intellectual capacity to appreciate that reality is a mixture of positivity and negativity.

It is extremely difficult to become aware of the shelter one lives in, of its precariousness, and of the way it structures one's life-world and one's relationships with other persons. One's shelter is a disposition that generates practices, beliefs, perceptions, feelings, and so forth. The task is to reveal and bring to light the active role that values play in holding together the patient's shelter and in shaping his abnormal and distressing experiences. This is the *via regia* that will help him to recalibrate his dysfunctional, miscarried position-taking and, finally, to recover his sense of responsibility and agency (Stanghellini, 2016a).

An example of a phenomenologically informed therapeutic values-based interview may be taken from the case of anorexia (Fulford and Stanghellini, forthcoming). The psychopathological core of the life-world of persons with anorexia nervosa is not feeling oneself in the first-person perspective, and in particular feeling extraneous to one's body and emotions. This entails a fleeting feeling of selfhood and an evanescent sense of identity (see Chapter 16). This vulnerable awareness of oneself is disturbing and generates the need to appraise oneself in alternative ways. One of the coping strategies or alternative means of self-recognition in these persons is feeling their body through the gaze of others. The Other has a key role in the life-world of persons with anorexia since it is through being looked at by others that these persons can achieve a feeling of their own body and a sense of identity. Obviously, this coping strategy is not voluntarily adopted and remains largely unconscious. A second way to regain a sense of identity is identifying oneself through one's passion for thinness as passions represent a rupture in the fleeting character of one's emotional and bodily life. The ossification of this passion and of the related value is the expression of the need to compensate the disturbing, shameful, and anxiogenic fleeting sense of selfhood and identity.

The unfolding (P) of the life-world of persons with anorexia and the analysis of their value-structure and position-taking (H) is essential if we want to demonstrate that it is a mistake to see these persons' values as merely imperfect cognition or as a kind of irrational or delusional belief about their body or nutrition. Rather, their values are a kind of religion that goes beyond the rationality/irrationality divide. It is about the worth of life and the way to make one's life meaningful. Food for them has a moral value: it is a sin and a temptation. Fatness and thinness – that is, one's bodily shape – have a moral value too. Fatness has a moral value as indicative of laziness, lack of self-care, and lack of self-control. Thinness means the capacity to give a shape to oneself and is more valuable than anything else including health and life itself. Strict rules are needed not to do wrong and to be led astray. Starvation is the unique salvation practice.

Dynamic Analysis (D)

The psycho-dynamic moment (D) of the PHD consists in tracing back the life-world (one's experiences and actions) and the world-view (one's values and position-taking) to the life-history in which they are embedded. To make sense of a given phenomenon is finally to posit it in a meaningful context, and this context includes the personal history of the patient.

With Binswanger (1928/1963) we call "personal life-history" the intimate interconnection of the contents of the person's experiences. Through histories (or narratives) we are able to articulate the reasons of our character and the meanings of the events that we encounter in our life. Narratives are patterns of meanings that contribute to make sense of my character and the *via regia* to work through the meaning of a given situation in my life. They moderate the ossification of character and the traumatic potential of the event. They make our involuntary dispositions and the alterity contained in the event a dynamic part of our personal history. The psycho-dynamic analysis consists, first of all, in the analysis of the *pathogenic situation*, that is, of the life situation that kindles the existential crisis and the psychopathological decomposition. Contrary to the standard notion of "trauma" which sees the person passively undergoing a distressing event, the notion of "situation" shows both the active (the person actively concurs in creating the situation) and the passive roles (the person does not consciously intend to create the situation) (Tellenbach, 1961/1980).

The pathogenic situation can be seen as a limit situation (Jaspers, 1925) in which the vulnerable structure of the patient is made manifest. Limit situations may turn into a pathogenetic situation when they impact a given existentially vulnerable person. Limit situations include vulnerability to guilt, inescapability of finitude, anxiety over freedom, fragility of one's body, loneliness of one's existence, etc.

The relation between pathogenetic situations and existentially vulnerable personality is a *key–lock relation* (Kretschmer, 1919) in the sense that each personality has its own specific limit situation. Fuchs offers some examples of such vulnerability: the hypochondriac's sensitivity to the perils of bodily existence, the anorexic's sensitivity to the dependency on a material body, the depressive's vulnerability in relation to freedom and guilt, and the narcissist's vulnerability to the limitation of possibilities (Fuchs, 2013c).

Existentially vulnerable persons establish themselves within the defensive walls of a shelter to avoid the contents uncovered by their specific limit situation (Fuchs, 2013c). For instance, for obsessive structures completeness and perfection are the basic assumption/housing that defends from contingency and unpredictability. For the melancholic type of personality (see Chapter 15) orderliness and hypernomia defend from guilt feelings. For the dependent personality hanging on to others is the way to avoid the anxiety of freedom. For the narcissistic personality continuously expanding one's status via success is a defense from finiteness, restriction, and imperfection.

The D moment of the PHD helps the patient to recognize her own limit situation and its implications, to accept it and to take a stance towards it. Limit situations thus uncover the basic conditions of existence, that is, being at risk of failure, guilt, death, financial ruin, etc. Personality structures are housings or shelters meant to defend from these threats. Yet these housings are precarious, vulnerable. The analysis of the pathogenic situation thus leads to the analysis of the patient's *vulnerable structure*. This indicates a significant combination of stable characteristics that make up the ontological constitution around which the vulnerability of the person is organized. A person's vulnerable structure is the amalgamation of a certain set of values and beliefs that serve as a protection from this person's limit situation. For instance, *antagonomia* in persons with schizophrenia, that is, their claiming one's independence as the most important value, can be seen as a shelter or defensive structure against their feeling of being vulnerable to the influx coming from the external world since for them conventional (common-sense) assumptions, social-shared knowledge, common ways of thinking and behaving, and immediate (empathic) relationships and emotional attunement are evaluated as dangerous sources of loss of individuation (see Chapter 14). The D moment of the PHD can lead a patient to understand their own shelter, its basic assumptions or philosophy of life, as a fragile defense against their own limit situation, and to the awareness of the failure of all attempts at solutions through such housings.

The analyses of the pathogenic situation and of the vulnerable structure are part and parcel of psycho-dynamics as the basic presuppositions of psycho-dynamics are psychological (existential) continuity and psychological determinism. The former assumes that all of the events in a person's life (including those that look inconsistent) are "lawful" and potentially meaningful in a particular way for that person. The latter assumes that all events in a person's life have at least as one of their causes a psychological cause and can thereby be explained on a psychological basis. The PHD method (Figure 11.1) endorses the first assumption, but only partially the second. The purpose of the D moment in the PHD method is not an archaeology, that is, the rescuing of a remote cause that is posited in the past (Stanghellini, 2016a). The psycho-dynamic process is not the search for a *big bang*. What is searched for is not a datum, an event that has taken place at the origin of a person's story. Rather, it is a phenomenon that allows the intelligibility of the other historical phenomena. It is something that belongs to a

P: Unfolding the patient's style of experience and action (life-world)

H: Illuminating the patient's value-structure and position-taking (world-view)

D: Grasping the patient's specific pathogenic situation and *Urphänomen* (life-history)

Figure 11.1 The PHD method

person's life-history that helps make intelligible a string of phenomena whose association might have passed unobserved. This something enforces the coherence and synchronic comprehensibility of the system (Agamben, 2008: 93). Looking into a person's past has not the purpose of finding a remote traumatic event that causally explains (to explain technically means *scire per causas*) the following events that have taken place. Rather, the purpose is looking for the phenomenon that can lend coherence to the person's life-history.

In the case of Giacomo, we may suppose that this phenomenon – we may call it the *Urphänomen* (original phenomenon) – is the very appearance of a garden in the mildest season of the year as the garden of universal souffrance. We can imagine that when he entered the garden, full of plants, herbs, and flowers, he realized with surprise that in every part he looked he found suffering. The sun does not give life to the rose, rather it makes it wrinkle, languish, wilt; a bee does not transmit life from one lily to the other, rather it cruelly sucks from its most sensitive, vital parts.

The *Urphänomen* is not chronologically original, but hermeneutically so. It may not be a traumatic event that has taken place in the remote past and gave origin to a given personal development. The *Urphänomen* is better understood as the best examplar of a class of phenomena that exhibits, shows, and points out the essential properties of that kind of phenomena. When Giacomo tells us his vision of the garden, we realize that this is the best exemplar of a group of analogous experiences whose common-sense significance is life and vitality, but which are appropriated by Giacomo as the emblem of cruelty and decay. For its transparency and completeness, the appearance of the garden as the emblem of death can help to illuminate all the other similar experiences Giacomo had in his life, according to the rule "one speaks for many." It is a single phenomenon in a person's life-history that being very perspicuous in its singularity can make intelligible an entire group of phenomena, whose semantic homogeneousness it has contributed to creating. If I discover the *Urphänomen* in a person's life-history, this will shed light on all other previously opaque phenomena by means of the analogy between itself and the other phenomena. The *Urphänomen* can transform a set of phenomena that, at face value, were unrelated into a *Gestalt* of meaningfully related phenomena.

To make this concept even clearer: the appearance of a garden in the mildest season of the year as the garden of universal souffrance is not a deeper symptom that generates surface symptoms, or a traumatic experience that generates other traumatic experiences. Rather, grasping it as the *Urphänomen* generates our own and the patient's capacity to make sense of other abnormal psychic phenomena. It is not an aetio-pathogenic construct, but rather a hermeneutic one. It can generate pathogenic or aetiological hypotheses, but it should not be taken as an aetio-pathogenic construct per se.

The supposed epistemological antinomy between meanings and causes, understanding and explaining, and between human and natural sciences is not at issue here. It can be assumed that meaningful motivations provide the fundamental lawfulness of mental life and act as causes for human behavior – *motivational causality*. It can also be assumed that the kind of information contained in motivations regulating behavior is encoded in states of the brain. The task of reconstructing the "causes" of human behavior in all cases is based on and must therefore be preceded – especially in a therapeutic context – by that of reconstructing its meaning which is encoded in the brain and motivates behavior. Thus, this task is first and foremost hermeneutical in nature.

Chapter

12

A Decalogue for the Therapeutic Interview

(1) Focusing on the patient's subjective experience (rather than mere behavior) as the point of departure of any clinical encounter.

(2) Encouraging the patient to unfold his experiences and make explicit his emotions and values as the core of his life-world and his personal horizon of meaning.

(3) Helping the patient to reflect upon his experiences, express them in a narrative format, and identify a core meaning, or meaning-organizer, around which his narrative can become meaningful for him.

(4) Supporting the patient in taking a position in front of the way he narrates and makes sense of his experiences.

(5) The clinician makes explicit to the patient his own experiences elicited by the patient's narratives, and his own understanding of the patient's narrative (assumptions, personal experiences, beliefs) as if it were his own.

(6) Through this process, the clinician also makes his own set of theoretical assumptions, personal experiences, values and beliefs, explicit.

(7) The clinician promotes a reciprocal exchange of perspectives with his patient.

(8) Clinician and patient cooperate in the co-construction of a new meaningful narrative that includes and, if possible, integrates contributions from both the original perspectives.

(9) The clinician tolerates diversity and potential conflicts of values and beliefs.

(10) Finally, the clinician facilitates coexistence when it is not possible to establish consensus.

2 Life-Worlds

Introduction

The aim of the therapeutic interview is to improve our *understanding* of the form of life incarnated by people suffering from mental disorders. This kind of understanding entails two basic moves. First, unfolding the patient's subtle and pervasive changes in the way he or she experiences and acts. Second, grasping the emotions and the personal values that subtend the patient's experiences and actions.

The first move consists in an in-depth, tactful, and empathic exploration of the patient's life-world, including the way he perceives his own body, self, others, space, time, etc. These experiences may be fleeting, perhaps even verging on something ineffable. Also, many patients may consider their experiences to be uniquely private. Clinicians should use their knowledge about these subtle experiential changes to help their patients find a language to communicate them and establish through this an authentic therapeutic alliance.

In this part of the book we provide a cartography of the life-world which persons affected by certain mental disorders live in, and the emotional atmosphere and value-structure in which their experience is enmeshed. These "maps" of prototypical psychopathological life-worlds will contribute to improve our resources for the therapeutic interview. Such a detailed knowledge of the experiential dimension of mental pathology will also develop our theoretical tools for valid and reliable diagnosis.

Some clinical situations can be enveloped in a quite inexplicable and ineffable atmosphere. In these situations theoretical knowledge is not enough and the clinical encounter is more like an aesthetic experience than an exchange of information between the interviewee and the interviewer based on the value of objectivity. The significance of atmospheres in clinical diagnosis and the importance of emotional intelligence for the success of the clinical encounter have long been established. Tellenbach (1968) considered that when interacting with a psychotic patient one feels a certain atmospheric quality, something that exceeds the factual and remains unsaid. Hence he developed the concept of "diagnostic atmosphere." Minkowski (1933/1970) talked about *diagnostique par pénétration* (diagnosis through penetration). It is often through the atmosphere into which we are initially thrown that we apprehend a given situation. This atmosphere is a kind of mood in which we are embedded. We sense this mood before we can make sense of it, long before we can establish a valid and reliable diagnosis. The fundamental way of being situated in the world is being in a given feeling-state or emotional tonality. Emotions are the primordial medium in which we are situated: this is true both for the patient and for the clinician. The sharing of an emotional atmosphere is the root of the genuine interpersonal communication (Buytendjik, 1988). Through atmospheres one is placed in a situation. This place is determined by a sense of proportion and distance, that preserves the sphere of the Other. The sense that orients us in an atmospheric encounter with the Other is *tact*: a special sensitivity and sensitiveness to situations and how to behave in them for which knowledge from general principles does not suffice. The capacity to say something tactfully is dependent on the capacity to sense an atmosphere.

Next to an in-depth awareness of the emotions permeating the clinical encounter, a precise knowledge of the patient's values is also fundamental. This will help not to conflate the patient's values with abnormal or delusional beliefs. Beliefs that depart from common sense are not *ipso facto* delusions. To conflate idiosyncratic values with delusions is not only conceptually wrong and ethically inadmissible, it is also therapeutically ineffective. Values are not symptoms to be "killed." They need modulation, therapeutic accommodation with the requirements of reality, not eradication.

Carefully assessing the patient's way of being in the world and of being with others, their emotions, and values is instrumental in projecting tailor-made therapeutic and rehabilitation programs, which should not only acknowledge the patient's skills, but also respect his or her principles, overall aims, and philosophy of life. A fine-grained knowledge about the way patients experience other persons and conceptualize interpersonal relationships is an essential prerequisite to establish an effective therapeutic relationship. It is a resource in modulating distance in the therapeutic interview, especially when we meet a patient in an early stage of his or her disorder, during which it is essential to avoid stigmatization, social isolation, and the person's identification with the role of the patient. It may help the patient to give his or her symptoms a format, to facilitate the unfolding of symptoms, and the capacity of the patient to take a reflexive stance over them.

The challenge facing the clinician is how to offer the patient an insight into her strange and disturbing experiences, as well as helping her to acquire the appropriate means to make sense and cope with her unease. The phenomenological character of the approach provides a theoretical framework to assess and explore the patient's experience of troubled personhood. This is an important methodological contribution to therapy, since it is open to an unusual extent in that it reveals aspects of experience that other approaches tend to overwrite or eclipse with their strong theoretical – and sometimes moralistic – claims. In this sense, we can say that the ethics of this approach is based on the principle of letting the patient have her say. The hermeneutical character of this approach provides a framework with room for the ethical problems involved in being a person who faces the metamorphosis of her own life-world. This principle admonishes the clinician to bracket her own prejudices and let the features of a pathological condition emerge in their peculiar feel, meaning, and value for the patient, thus making every effort to focus on the patient's suffering as experienced and narrated by her.

Chapter

13

The Life-World of Borderline Persons

Borderline personality disorder (BPD) is a highly variegated clinical constellation of abnormal phenomena characterized by unstable mood, behavior, and relationships. It represents the most diagnosed condition, in particular in the last few years. Despite different approaches that tend to emphasize different aspects of BPD, there is a general agreement about the fact that its principal features are the following: (1) emotions tend to be intense and rapidly shifting; (2) relationships tend to be conflicted and stormy; (3) there may be impulsive, self-destructive, or self-defeating behaviors; and (4) there is a lack of a clear and coherent sense of identity. Indeed, borderline people are often described as affected by extreme emotional fluctuations and by the sudden emergence of uncontrollable and disproportionate emotional reactions. They often appear deprived of a stable sense of identity and unable to be steadily involved in a given life project or social role.

In this chapter, we describe BPD from the angle of the emotions displayed by these persons. In particular, we focus in great detail on dysphoria and anger, the main emotions characterizing borderline persons. We assume that their existence oscillates between dysphoria and anger: dysphoric mood is a permanent trait, and angry affect is an intermittent state. We also describe despair, boredom, shame, and guilt, which represent other fundamental emotions affecting borderline persons and accompanying dysphoria and anger.

We also assume that dysphoria and anger generate two different life-worlds to borderline persons since each emotion situates a person, disclosing a determinate set of possibilities for experience and action. Thus, our descriptions of the borderline life-world will include two distinct configurations: the dysphoric life-world and the life-world of anger. The world of dysphoria is characterized by a painful experience of incoherence and inner emptiness, a feeling of uncertainty and inauthenticity in interpersonal relationships, and an excruciating sense of futility and inanity of life. But it also entails a sense of vitality, although a disorganized, aimless, and explosive one. In the world of anger the vague and confused sense of self and others is suddenly replaced by a clear, although elementary normative, universe in which it is painfully obvious to the borderline person who is "good" (oneself) and who is "bad" (the other). This sudden feeling of infallible rightness helps the borderline person to find his lost identity in a world that momentarily regains its structure and meaning.

Emotions are also tightly linked to the values and norms by means of which we orient ourselves in the world and represent other people and ourselves. In the third section of this chapter we will make a comprehensive analysis of the value-structure of persons with BPD. As we explained in Chapter 8, emotions are what make us care about the conventions, rules, values, and norms that structure and orient our experience of the world, other people, and ourselves (De Sousa, 2011). This is not to say that values and norms are merely emotional.

On the contrary, values, and norms in particular, are the more stable, i.e. less emotion-dependent, points of orientation that enable us to distance ourselves from what we may feel in a given situation (Blackburn, 1998).

Emotions in Borderline Persons

Emotions are the core of a person's life-world, or the spatializing-temporalizing vortex that situates a person (Merleau-Ponty, 1945/1962), allowing that person to perceive the things that surround him as disclosing certain (and not other) possibilities for experience and action. Borderline persons have serious emotional problems. They have very intense baseline emotions and a tendency to respond to life-events and environmental triggers with unusually strong emotions. They rapidly shift from one emotion to another, and have serious problems in regulating them. Emotional dysregulation and instability are considered a trait dimension, a vulnerability feature underlying BPD, present before the onset of symptoms (Stanghellini and Rosfort, 2013a).

Anger and Dysphoria

There are two basic emotions characterizing the life-world of borderline persons: *anger* and *dysphoria*. As we have seen in Chapter 8, there are two kinds of emotions: affects and moods. The former are focused and possess a specific directedness, whereas the latter are unfocused and do not possess a specific directedness and aboutness. In this perspective, anger is an affect and dysphoria is a mood. With this in place, we shall try to pinpoint the main characteristics of anger and dysphoria.

Anger is an emotion usually triggered by a personal offense, or having been somehow wronged by another person, and as such it often motivates a desire for retaliation. Anger shares with rage and fury their connection with assaultive behavior which summons these affects as a sinister shadow. Despite its complex cognitive, personal, and social aspects (Solomon, 2007), anger is, in most cases, a readily identified emotion because of its rather clear behavioral manifestations such as increase of muscle tension, scowling, grinding of teeth, glaring, clenching of fists, changes of arm position and body posture, flushing and paling (Tavris, 1989). Anger and aggressive behaviors (as we will see in great detail) characterize the acute phases of the borderline person's existence.

The psychological and psychopathological characterization of *dysphoria*, on the other hand, requires more attention because of its more subdued manifestation and less direct connection to behavioral patterns. Dysphoria manifests itself as a prolonged, unmotivated, indistinct, and quasi-ineffable constellation of feelings that convey a nebula of vague impulses, sensations, and perceptions that permeate a person's whole field of awareness. The psychological and psychopathological characterization of dysphoria is quite difficult because of its subdued manifestation and loose connection to behavioral patterns. The word "dysphoria" derives from the ancient Greek δύσφορος (dysphoros), formed as δυσ- (dis-), difficult, and φέρω (phero), to bear. It is an oppressive, and sometimes unbearable, mood. So, even in its etymological roots the word "dysphoria" is quite polysemous, nearly overlapping "bad mood" in very general terms, vaguely defining an emotional condition in which a person is heavily oppressed, and in which that person may either react and show his feelings, or passively suffer and submit to them (Stanghellini, 2000a; Stanghellini and Rosfort, 2013a, 2013b). Phenomenal characterizations of dysphoria mainly focus on its being felt as a burden one cannot get rid of because it is not external to one's own self. It is an obstacle to movement and, at the same time, it may generate impatience, restlessness, and an incoercible impulse to move away without a definite goal. It is also experienced as an uncomfortable feeling characterized by being both painful and sorrowful, as well as discontented and indignant. This complexity elicits opposite kinds of movement such as inaction/action, resignation/resistance, suffering/retaliation (Stanghellini and Rosfort, 2013a, 2013b). Also, in dysphoria, the normal distinction between self and other is blurred and hazy.

Furthermore, it has a horizontal absorption in the sense that it attends to the world as a whole, not focusing on any particular object or situation. No particular action is dictated by dysphoric mood. On the contrary, it complicates the relation between feeling and action because it introduces doubt, hesitation, and questions. The intentional structure that characterizes much of human emotional experience is absent in dysphoria. In other words, dysphoric mood is (to use Kimura's 2000 terminology) pure *noesis* or *noematically empty* intentionality. With "noesis" we mean a mental act (e.g. an act of perception), whereas with "noema" we mean the mental object to which this act is addressed (e.g. a representation). Dysphoria is a mood that consists of a purely noetic act without a representational or linguistic target. Noematic representations function as a dispositive "to control the noetic act so that it does not deviate from its relationship with life" (Kimura, 2000: 88; our translation). This characterization tallies perfectly with the experience that borderline persons have of their own dysphoric mood: an untamed source of vitality, a disturbing and an exuberant force, creative and destructive at the same time, a vigor that brings life as well as annihilation. We will come back to this characterization of dysphoria as *desperate vitality* in detail in the section on the dysphoric life-world.

In the borderline person's existence there is a dialectic between dysphoria and anger:

- Dysphoria is a *permanent trait*. We can identify a dysphoric emotional complex that includes dysphoria, irritability, internal agitation, and emotional lability. This is the *background mood trait* characterizing persons with BPD (Stanghellini and Rosfort, 2013a). It is the long-lasting and profound emotional tonality or basic temperament in which the borderline person is enmeshed, and as such it influences both the voluntary and involuntary aspect of her perceptions and actions. The existence of borderline persons exhibits prolonged states dominated by dysphoric mood. This emotional state is saturated with a brimming constellation of feelings without any explicit object or target, a state of tension that may lead to spontaneously vigorous outbursts as well as to pale stagnation or emotional depletion.

- Anger is an *acute intermittent state*. Intermittently, borderline persons enter acute episodes of excitement in which anger may prevail. Anger is the affective state that punctuates the existence of the borderline person. Angry outbursts, emanating from the dysphoric background, are typically accompanied by feelings of shame and humiliation and may generate acute micro-psychotic episodes during which the borderline person may develop paranoid symptoms, including transitory delusion-like and hallucination-like phenomena. Persecutory delusions may develop out of these episodes, in which the persecutor is typically a significant other (the patient's partner, relative, or therapist, for example).[1]

---

[1] It is necessary, about this aspect, to eliminate some possible misunderstandings. All types of delusions or delusion-like ideas occurring in borderline persons have an ontic, rather than ontological, character. They are about the basic concerns that characterize our daily existence,

- Dysphoria can also be an *acute intermittent state*. Alternatively, the person may collapse into acute episodes during which their dysphoric mood exacerbates, culminating in a painful paralysis of action characterized by feelings of spleen, boredom, despair, emptiness, dissatisfaction; or in other words, a mixture of, or a rapid oscillation between, dysphoric mood and more focused affects like disgust, fear, and occasionally anger (concerning oneself or others). This may entail tormenting ideas of meaninglessness, persecutory guilt, and, in the most severe cases, suicidal ideation.

There are other emotions that may have a special importance in the experience of border-line persons, namely, *boredom, shame*, and *guilt*. Since they are extremely important to understand the borderline's life-world they need to be described in separate paragraphs.

Boredom

Boredom is a mood characterized by a pervasive lack of interest in everything. The entire world is monotonous, and this monotonousness cannot be analyzed by the person into further elements, but encloses their surroundings, things as well as persons, in a vague and unarticulated way: the world as a whole "seeps towards me from the globe like a cosmic fog, deadening my mind, slackening my will, and depleting me of energy" (Smith, 1986: 191). A helpful way to describe an emotion is to illustrate the scenario this emotion brings about. This means that each emotion implies a given configuration of the surrounding world and a given movement by the person who is affected by that emotion. In this vein, and drawing from Smith's account, we can say that boredom flows forwards, towards me in a dulling manner. Not violently or sharply, but slowly and languorously.[2] I flow backwards in a dulled manner, wearied and blunted by the monotony of the whole. While bored, the world-whole is just happening and is blank – a blankness that endures. Lived space is an indifferent extension, devoid of salience, offering no directions, moribund. It conveys a feeling of meaninglessness and *finis vitae*. Lived time is an oppressing stillness. One's movements remain stuck in indecisiveness. The other is distant, meaningless, annoying.

Heidegger (2001) recognizes three form of boredom: (1) becoming bored *with* some-thing (or be sick of something) (*Gelangweiltwerden von etwas*), (2) being bored *by* some-thing (*Sichlangweilen bei etwas*), and (3) profound boredom (*tiefe Langweile*). Each form of boredom is distinguished from the others in terms of its relation to how time passes (see also Freeman and Elpidorou, 2015).

The first form of boredom is the most familiar – what we might identify with our pre-theoretical understanding of boredom – but for Heidegger, it is also the most trivial. It occurs when we are bored with some person, object, or state of affairs that causes annoyance. As we all know, being bored is unpleasant. When we experience it, we try to make the time pass by distracting ourselves. Very often though, our attempts to get rid of

---

including our fears of being abandoned and mistreated, and for the way we appear to others and their opinion about what kind of person we are. This brings the kind of delusions exhibited by borderline persons very close to those that are typical in other *affective* psychoses, like melancholia (i.e. psychotic depression, where the main themes are moral guilt, impoverishment, and hypochondria) and mania (delusions of grandeur like genealogical and mystical ones). Borderline persons are deluded about reality, whereas schizophrenic persons are deluded about the reality of reality (Stanghellini, 2008).

[2] Interestingly, in English "bore" also means a high steep-fronted wave moving up a narrow estuary, caused by a tide.

boredom are in vain. This form of boredom arises, quoting Heidegger's example, while waiting at the station for our train which has been delayed, and because there is a lack of communication we don't know when the train is going to arrive. Being bored with something is characterized by two aspects that are intimately related to one another: it leaves us empty and holds us in limbo. This kind of boredom leaves us empty because it fails to offer us any fulfillment: what we find at the station, for example, does not engage us nor does it promote our interests. It holds us in limbo because, when one is bored, time drags along. Consequently, that which will bring us fulfillment is postponed: in this case, boarding the train, arriving at our destination, and, for example, seeing our loved ones.

The second form of boredom is both more profound and slightly more complicated than the first. Whereas in the first form of boredom there is an intentional object known to the person who is bored, that is, a situation or a person who is boring, in this form of boredom, *there is no determinate person or object that is boring*. Rather, what we are bored with is something indeterminate and unfamiliar: something that has the character of "I know not what" (Heidegger, 2001: 172), and that Heidegger ultimately identifies with the passing of time itself – not in the form of time dragging, as in the first form of boredom, but rather in the sense of *time standing still*. Heidegger's example of this form of boredom is attending a dinner party, on our own volition, and in an attempt to kill time. At the party, the food, company, and music are all pleasant. Indeed, "[t]here is nothing at all to be found that might have been boring about this evening ... Thus we come home quite satisfied" (Heidegger, 2001: 165). And yet, when we reflect upon the evening and situate it in terms of what was interrupted in order to attend the party and of what is coming in the next days, it dawns on us that we were bored all this time after all. Importantly, and unlike the first form of boredom, in this case, boredom "arises from out of *Dasein* itself" (Heidegger, 2001: 193). It is on account of our comportment towards the evening that boredom arises. Our own decision to partake in such a predictable, and *in retrospect* dull, event results in an emptiness: the party does not fulfill us. Thus, the second form of boredom, just like the first one, is also characterized by the fact that it leaves us empty. But unlike the first one, which has a rather clear intentional object from the outset (I am annoyed by the train's delay when I'm waiting for it), the second form of boredom has a *post hoc* intentional object, that is, the person feels bored not during the party, but when the party is over and he reconsiders and re-evaluates the party as a useless waste of time. We could also say that, whereas in the first form of boredom we do not feel responsible for the waste of time, in the second we feel guilty for the wrong decision that made us waste our time and forget our projects and interests.

The reason for this can be explained as follows: in terms of temporality, our decision to attend the party and to become absorbed by it has modified our having been and future: in a sense, we have forgotten them both. As a result, time appears to stand still: not insofar as it drags on and oppresses us (as it did in the first form of boredom), but rather insofar as our very existential present (the manner in which entities are disclosed to us) is cut off from our past (thrownness) and from our future (projection). This second form of boredom is more profound than the first: not only does it arise out of *Dasein* itself, but it also reveals an inauthentic modification of our temporal existence.

Profound boredom is the third and deepest form of boredom. It is an extreme and overwhelming experience in which everything bores us and unlike the first form of boredom, there is no point in fighting it. In profound boredom we stand without any concerns and interests. Profound boredom strips away all identifying characteristics, history, or projects; beings as a whole withdraw, and as with anxiety, they lose all significance. In profound boredom, absolute indifference overtakes us and we become insignificant as all things. This form of boredom thus renders us "an undifferentiated no one" by disclosing to us a world with no meaning or significance (Heidegger, 2001: 203). Profound boredom, like the other two forms of boredom, leaves us empty. But the emptiness in this case is more profound. Nothing matters to us. Nothing attracts us. There is nothing to which we can relate.

In the borderline existence, the kind of boredom implicated is the third form mentioned by Heidegger. Here, boredom is central among the feelings involved in the dysphoric mood. It shares with dysphoria the same temporal structure (monotonousness) and an analogous feeling of bluntness. Indeed, in boredom as well as in dysphoria the world, other people, and oneself just happen and are void of significance.

The disappearance of meaning and significance that people with BPD experience in boredom is correlated with temporality. Total indifference means not only that everything around us (or alongside of ourselves) has been drained of meaning (Heidegger, 2001: 215–217). It also means that nothing carries future prospects for us and that nothing relates and gives meaning to our past. But such a total withdrawal of beings is possible, Heidegger contends, only if *Dasein* "can no longer go along with them," if it is "entranced," and if its originary temporality has been modified (Heidegger, 2001: 221). Indeed, in borderline boredom, all three temporal dimensions of *Dasein* (past, present, and future) blend together and it is this "unarticulated unity" that entrances *Dasein* (Heidegger, 2001: 222). What bores us is not any specific entity or state of affairs; rather, it is time (as originary temporality) itself. Time bores us by entrancing and binding us. So, in this way, the mind goes blank. Nothing has a sense. The person with BPD goes around in circles, and in a purposeless way. They are without aim in life or more precisely, they cannot grasp the possibilities of becoming.

Shame

Whereas boredom is a mood that stymies my mind and dulls my attention, *shame*, on the other hand, is an affect that awakens and focuses my attention. When I feel ashamed, I am aware of being seen by another person whose gaze uncovers a part of who I am, usually a part that makes me feel embarrassed, inadequate, dishonored, and humiliated (Stanghellini and Rosfort, 2013a, 2013b). Shame has a sensation flow of suddenly and sharply falling downwards, an unpleasant and unwelcome experience that disposes me unfavorably towards the source of humiliation. The source of humiliation (the Other) is in a dominant position, growing bigger and bigger as I sink downwards. Lived space in shame has a centripetal character as one experiences a feeling of centrality. I feel my body naked, deprived of any protection, dirtied, soiled. The Other is in a dominant position, a watcher or a witness. Lived time comes to a fixation in an instant that grows to infinity. My identity is constantly threatened by the instability brought about by humiliation.

The effect of shame is that it reduces the complexity of the person that I am to one single aspect of it: when I feel ashamed, I know that for the Other I am *nothing but* that specific feature of the complexities of who I am. In shame, I feel that *I* (i.e. my whole self) disappear, while that detail – the *stain* – of myself that made me feel ashamed is magnified, becomes over-conspicuous and gets the front-stage. Shame reveals to me my selfhood as an object for another; as Sartre writes: "Shame ... is shame of *self*; it is the *recognition* of the fact that I *am* indeed that object which the Other is looking at and judging. I can be ashamed only as my freedom escapes me in order to become a *given* object" (Sartre, 1943/1992: 261).

The other persons are piercing gazes that nail me to what awakened my feeling of shame, that is, something, like an act or an omission, or some failing or defect, which elicited contempt, derision, or avoidance from other people. Shame means to be utterly exposed to the present, to the painful presence of devaluing gazes, to annihilating disdain and contempt (Fuchs, 2002).

A comparison between shame and two cognate feelings – humility and modesty – can help to further characterize this emotion and to focus on its anthropological meaning.

Humility is a gentle and welcome feeling of lowering myself beneath a reality that I intuitively feel to be absolutely above me. Whereas reverence flows downwards and backwards in a deferential and respectful manner, humility does not flow backwards but only downwards. In humility I gaze down at myself. I feel the height, the loftiness of the other indirectly by experiencing the extent of my lowliness. Whereas humiliation and shame are painful, humility has a pleasurable quality. I want and deserve to put myself beneath this highest reality. I want to be in its intuitive presence.

Modesty is a self-protecting feeling whereby I conceal myself. Modesty is the "natural veil of the soul ... the envelop of the body" (Nietzsche, quoted in Scheler, 1928/2012: 23). Clothes are only a crystallization of modesty: Aphrodite is shown in the nude, yet, the veil of modesty covers her more than any garment could do. Her beauty and concealment in modesty are inter-contained and one. The essence of modesty is a revelation of beauty in the manner of concealing itself. ("Der Kern der Scham ist eine Offenbarung der Schonheit in der Geste ihres Sichverbergens," Scheler, 1928/2012: xix.)

We owe to Scheler the understanding of shame as the emotion that shows *man's position in the cosmos*. The feeling of shame belongs to the *clair-obscure* of human nature. For man's unique place within the structure of the world and its entities is between the divine and animality. It expresses itself nowhere so clearly and immediately as in the feeling of shame. At first glance its "location" appears to be the living contact which man's spirit (as the quintessence of all supra-animal or mental acts such as thinking, intuiting, willing, loving, and their form of existence, the "person") has with drive life and the feelings of life which differ only by degrees from those of other animals. Shame is the revelation of the nature of man: the basic condition for the feeling of shame to occur is only given when in man the light of consciousness is existentially bound up with the living organism and shines down on the inner life. Shame arises originally by way of the contiguity between higher levels of consciousness and lower drive-awareness. Shame is *guiltless guilt*: a specific form of this experience of opposites that appears to be the root of the dark and peculiar feeling of shame. It is always conjoined with an element of "astonishment," "confusion," and an experience between what ideally "ought to be" and what, in fact, is. In such a kind of experience is to be found the foundation of the thousands of forms of the idea of the "fall" of man in religious myth. And only because spiritual personhood is experienced as essentially independent of the "lived body" and of everything that comes from it, is it possible to get into the position where we can feel shame. In shame we can see the position of man as a "bridge" or "transition": "spirit" and "flesh," eternity and time, essence and existence touch one another in a peculiar and obscure manner. One feels in one's depths and knows oneself to be a "bridge," a "transition" between two orders of being in which one has such equally strong roots that one cannot sever them without losing one's very "humanity." Man must feel shame – not because of this or that "reason" and not because we can be ashamed "of" this or that. We must feel shame because of our being a continuous movement and a transition itself.

To the origin of the feeling of shame there belongs something like an imbalance and disharmony in man between the sense and the claim of spiritual personhood and embodied needs. It is only because the human essence is tied up with a "lived body" that we can get in the position where we must feel shame.

Guilt

Finally, *guilt* is a moral feeling that typically arises when we think that we have in some way wronged another person. As such, it is the fundamental theme in those forms of major depression affecting the melancholic type of personality.[3] Depressive episodes in borderline persons, though, are not characterized by guilt feeling. Another kind of delusional theme, similar to the one developed by the sensitive character, is sometimes called *persecutory guilt* (Grinberg, 1964). Grinberg explains that guilt is implicitly contained in all experience of loss. This theory is based on psychoanalytic observations and supported by the etymology of the English verb "to lose," deriving from Old English *losian* which means "to perish" as well as "to destroy," and Italian and French verbs *perdere* and *perdre*, deriving from Latin *perdo*. The proportion of guilt determines the persecutory or depressive taint in the experience of loss. Persecutory guilt is the delusional theme whereby the patient feels persecuted for a fault he believes himself to have really committed, and especially for the loss of his moral integrity. Persons who develop persecutory guilt exhibit a mixture of guilt and shame. They feel guilty for what they have done, for instance, if they believe they harmed another person, and ashamed, because they have fallen short of what they might have hoped of themselves (Stanghellini and Rosfort, 2013b). As Bernard Williams writes: "We can feel both guilt and shame towards the same action. In a moment of cowardice, we let someone down; we feel guilty because we have let them down, ashamed because we have contemptibly fallen short of what we might have hoped of ourselves. As always, the action stands between the inner world of disposition, feeling, and decision and an outer world of harm and wrong" (Williams, 1993: 92).

Immediately after describing this interrelation between guilt and shame, Williams goes on to remark that what I have done points in one direction towards what has happened to others, in another direction to what I am; in other words, guilt looks primarily in the direction of others, while shame affects my understanding of the person that I am. We will analyze in detail the issue of guilt in the section on the borderline person's values. Table 13.1 summarizes the differences between guilt and shame.

Emotional Complexes: Dysphoric vs. Melancholic Depression

To make sense of this tense dialectic between dysphoria and anger, we need to explain the peculiar vitality that is the principal feature distinguishing borderline depression from other kinds of depression.

---

[3] The concept of *typus melancholicus* (TM) was formed with the help of phenomenological analyses in order to describe the personality of endogenous depressives (Tellenbach, 1961/1980). In continental European and Japanese psychopathology, it has been instrumental to the understanding of major depressives' pre-morbid and inter-morbid lifestyle, social behaviours, values and beliefs, precipitating situations, and acute clinical pictures (Mundt et al., 1996).

Table 13.1 Guilt vs. shame

	Guilt	Shame
Cause	Action, omission	Action, omission, failing, defect
Sense	Hearing (judge's voice)	Sight (being seen)
Internalized Other (I.O.)	Victim	Watcher, witness
I.O.'s emotion	Anger, resentment, indignation (forgiveness)	Contempt, derision
One's emotion at the I.O.'s emotion	Fear of punishment (reparation)	Unprotectedness, loss of power/clothedness (reconstruct/improve oneself)
Self/World	Even if I disappeared guilt would come with me	Wish to hide/disappear
Directedness	Look towards what has happened to the other (other-directed)	Looks to what I am (inner-directed)

As we saw above, the borderline existence is characterized by a paradoxical nature of power, destructive and creative at the same time – a power that brings with it a desperate vitality. Indeed, borderline persons experience themselves and others as blurred and fragmented, which provokes excruciating feelings of incoherence, emptiness, uncertainty, and inauthenticity. At the same time, though, the borderline person shows spontaneous surges of vitality, although disorganized and aimless.

To eliminate some possible misunderstandings about the psychopathological and noso-logical status of depression in borderline persons, we need to contrast the type of depression in borderline persons with another prototypical form of major depression, namely melancholia (see Chapter 15 for details). If we strictly confine ourselves to *major depression* as it is defined in current diagnostic manuals, there are at least two types that must be kept separate. In a seminal paper, Gunderson and Philips (1991) contrasted "empty" depression, which affects persons with BPD, with "guilt" depressions that mirror more classical forms of mood disorders. Comparing a sample of patients with borderline personality disorder vs. non-borderlines, both developing a major depressive episode, Westen and Cohen (1993) confirmed that depression in borderline patients is characterized by emptiness, loneliness, and desperation in relation to attachment figures, together with labile, diffuse negative affectivity. The phenomenality of depression is "distinct in borderline patients, centering on concerns about abandonment and rejection, a sense of emptiness and meaninglessness, and a view of the self as fundamentally evil or despicable" (Westen and Cohen, 1993: 358). Obviously, these two types of depression do not cover the whole depressive spectrum. There are, for instance, forms of melancholic depression that do not have guilt (i.e. the loss of moral integrity) as their main theme, but are characterized more by hypochondriac and bankruptcy delusions (i.e. the loss of bodily and financial integrity). What is relevant, though, in the context of our argument is that we are witnessing a profound transformation of the clinical forms of depression: whereas in handbooks of psychiatry published until

30 years ago melancholia was the typical, if not the paradigmatic, form of depression (e.g. Mayer-Gross, Slater, and Roth, 1954; Ey, 1959; Ey, Bernard, and Brisset, 1960), in more recent times we have seen an epidemic of non-melancholic forms of "atypical" depression in which guilt, loss, and vital sadness are not the central phenomena, but rather a confusing mixture of emptiness, abandonment, persecution, restlessness, impulsivity, dysphoria, and anger.

Differences in emotional profile in borderline vs. melancholic depressions have also been empirically established. Compared to borderline patients who develop depressive episodes, melancholic patients show very low rates of anger and dysphoria. They complain about their lack of emotional resonance with other persons and the environment, and, most importantly, they feel guilty for this lack of emotional involvement. The depressive experience of borderline patients is imbued with a tense, irritated mood, feelings of emptiness, higher proneness to externalize anger, resentment towards the environment, relatively high reactivity to environmental solicitations, and usually low levels of guilt feelings (Stanghellini, Bertelli, and Raballo, 2006).

These empirical findings should allow us to seek out more nuanced differences between the two sets of abnormal phenomena. Depressed mood is a complex emotional state that includes at least the following features: feeling of prostration (as in lack of vital drive), loss of pleasure and interest (emotional anaesthesia), and moral pain. If each of these features is carefully considered we can recognize significant differences between the two major prototypes of depression in question.

In borderline depressions, rather than a feeling of diminished vitality, we find a threatening sense of uncontrollable energy that dissipates the person's sense of agency and may therefore end up in a sensation of complete exhaustion and prostration. We do not find an over-identification of oneself with one's own body. Rather, one's own body, as the source of vitality and drive, is felt as if out of voluntary control, lying somewhere between self and something which is not the self (*"Not a pleasant energy, rather an uncomfortable feeling of excess"*). In borderline depression the body is experienced as charged with an energy that does not seem to belong to oneself, that is, it disrupts a person's sense of being a self by transforming that person's body into an anonymous source of vitality (*"Something biting, scorching, burning, I don't know"*).

With regard to anhedonia (another peculiar characteristic of melancholia), when it appears in borderline persons as a feature of a depressive episode, it typically consists in a kind of irritating emptiness that oscillates between painful feelings of abandonment and self- and other-destructive actings-out, including a mixture of anger and humiliation. If this emptiness is to be understood as some form of anhedonia, it is certainly very different from the kind of anhedonia that we find in melancholic depression, since the borderline's feelings of emptiness are more akin to an overcharged, hypersensitive, and frustrated emotional resonance – as if it consisted of raw feelings that blunt the emotional life because of their unmediated intensity.

Furthermore, depressive episodes in borderline persons are not characterized by this kind of guilt feeling. Typical borderline persons think that they suffer because they *have been wronged* by the other person. Guilt is on the side of the other – usually a significant other. Sometimes, though, borderline persons are also affected by a moral pain that has been called "persecutory guilt" (Grinberg, 1964). Persecutory guilt is the delusional theme whereby the patient feels persecuted for a fault she senses she has really committed, though without being explicitly aware of being responsible for her fault. To explain this point, we need to distinguish two different emotional complexes involving moral pain: one is characterized by a constellation of guilt, humiliation, and anger; the other by guilt, shame, and remorse. This first complex is typical in borderline depression, whereas the second can be found in melancholic depression.

While the feelings of guilt involved in melancholic patients tend to evoke shame when thinking about the wronged other, persecutory guilt is characterized by a feeling of being humiliated by the other with regard to oneself. Also, guilt and shame in melancholic patients are self-referential: they feel guilty and ashamed in front of themselves. Persecutory guilt and humiliation in borderline patients involve the other: they feel wronged and humiliated by the other, whose *look* is responsible for revealing to everybody their faults and for laying bare "petty" moral flaws in their character.

Another important feature that can help to disentangle borderline from melancholic depression is the kind of limit situation that generates each of them. Normally, melancholic depression is triggered by experiences of *loss*, which the patient construes as *her own* wrong behavior, whereas the borderline person is sensible to experiences of *abandonment*, which she construes as wrong behavior on the part of *the other person*. For borderline persons, other people oscillate between opposite polarities: a hoped-for source of selfhood through recognition, but also of humiliation and thus of disunion and despair. Shame is born from frozen unresolved traumatic experiences of non-recognition. Shame and feeling humiliated, unvalued, and unworthy reach a fever pitch when they are triggered by what seems to others to be insignificant actions or words. It takes one negative feeling or thought to trigger a landslide of negative feelings and thoughts. Unable to cope with the quickly escalating pain, borderline persons often act out or experience rage, or if they feel a great amount of anxiety they may be demanding, needy, and clinging (Bradshaw, 1994).

The Life-Worlds of Persons with Borderline Personality Disorder

We have described in detail anger and dysphoria, the main emotions characterizing borderline persons. As we saw above, dysphoria is empty intentionality, so to speak, devoid of the moderating power of language and representation. Dysphoria exerts a centrifugal force which fragments the borderline person's representations of herself and of others, inducing a painful experience of incoherence and inner emptiness, a feeling of uncertainty and inauthenticity in interpersonal relationships, and an excruciating sense of futility and inanity of life. But it also entails a sense of vitality, although a disorganized, aimless, and explosive one – a desperate vitality.

On the other hand, anger is an emotion normally conceived as involving a personal offense, or having been somehow wronged by another person, and as such it often motivates a desire for retaliation. Anger may restore the cohesion of the self, determine a clear-cut, unambiguous image of the other person, and dissipate all doubts and sentiments of absurdity – at the cost, however, of representing the other as unambiguously menacing. Anger tends to preserve and maintain a precarious cohesion of the self (Pazzagli and Rossi Monti, 2000), in the sense that venting one's anger is a way of feeling alive and of affirming one's right to exist as the unique person that one is. In anger episodes, the vague and confused sense of values and norms that characterizes borderline existence is suddenly replaced by a crystal clear, although elementary normative, universe in which it is painfully obvious to the borderline person who is "good" (oneself) and who is "bad" (the other). This sudden feeling of infallible rightfulness helps the borderline person to find his or her lost identity in a world that momentarily regains its structure and meaning. This emotional complex (dysphoria and anger) engenders very different kinds of existential orientation and enactment, thereby enacting very different configurations of being-in-the-world, entailing the metamorphosis of the life-world that borderline persons live in.

To put it more sharply, dysphoria and anger are the "psychopathological organizers" (Rossi Monti and Stanghellini, 1996) of the life-worlds borderline persons live in, conferring both unitary and clear meaning to the heterogeneousness of the pathological phenomena characterizing borderline existence.

In the following, we analytically illustrate the basic structures of the dysphoric life-world and of the life-world of anger.

The Life-World of Dysphoria

Time

There are two main time features to the life-world of dysphoria. The first is *monotonousness*. Time can be experienced as a tedious, wearing, dull cloud in which past, present, and future are not clearly separable. The second is *instantaneousness*. Time is experienced as an absolute "now" into which the person, her identity, and history collapse.

We have seen this first feature of borderline temporality while describing profound boredom. In profound boredom one feels stripped away from all identifying characteristics, history, or projects. It renders one "an undifferentiated no one" and discloses a world with no meaning or significance. In boredom, as well as in dysphoria, nothing matters to us, nothing attracts us, there is nothing to which we can relate. The world, other people, and oneself just happen and are void of significance.

To the borderline person, the "now" is *pure presentification*, lacking extension into the future (*protention*) and into the past (*retention*). Presenting themselves independently from past and future, they cannot feel the "length" of these nows, as it is possible with a present that develops out of the past and is directed towards the future. Each now moment thus becomes an infinity that in some sense "communicates with eternity" (Kimura, 1992: 150). This kind of absolute "now" has no temporal delimitation, no historical determination, and no linguistic-symbolic articulation. This isolated, ineffable, and absolute "now" is not able to carry any kind of relation to, or become an integrated part of, the narrative identity of the borderline person. In these moments, an acute feeling of despair, i.e. discordant directions of intentionality leading to a paralysis of thinking and action, accompanies dysphoria. The present moment, lived as an absolute now, lacks depth, value, and existential meaning (for details see "Narrative Self and Limit Situation" section). This "transitory present has no depth. It lacks the fulfillment which only originates from the integration of past experience and anticipated future" (Fuchs, 2007: 381).

Yet in the life-world of dysphoria the absorption in the present moment quite paradoxically does not just convey feelings of void and monotonousness, but also thrilling experiences of instantaneousness. Time in the life-world of dysphoria is punctuated by "islands of feast" in a stagnant "ocean of spleen." It is being "dead for a long time" (Kane, 2001: 214) interrupted by transient, vanishing, volatile moments of intensity. Boredom is punctuated with moments of excitement, thrill, during which one's blind vitality finds its fulfillment. This side of time experience in persons affected by BPD is called by Bin Kimura (1992) *intra festum*. As in the atmosphere of a feast, here we find the irruption of spontaneity and ecstasy, oblivious of the past and the future. Blind spontaneity is the opposite of voluntary autonomy as the rapture of ecstasy is the opposite of engaged care. Moreover, borderline persons are unable to cope with the flux of immediateness, and this flux becomes paroxysmal, and immediateness chaotic. The borderline person, immersed in the *intra festum*, is characterized by a short-circuit of selfhood in front of the paroxysm of chaotic immediateness. The absolute "now" is the night of the self and the disintegration of personhood, since continuity in time is fundamental for a self to be an integral part of the person that she is. Kimura suggests that in borderline temporality there is no separation, no space in between the "now" and the person: the person collapses into its "now" (Stanghellini and Rosfort, 2013a, 2013b).

Thus, the present moment is *momentary* in the sense that it is lived as evanescent, fast, fugaceous, and fleeting. But next to this volatile and empty character of temporality, sometimes the events that happen to the dysphoric person are not just momentary, but also *momentous*, that is, overwhelmingly significant to him. The present moment can be spasmodic, urgent, clamant: e.g. *"When my telephone rings, it's him; it's imperative to me, I cannot escape from it," "Time is pressing me, I must seize the moment," "Time is clamant, opportunities come rarely and call me with a loud voice," "Doc, I need to see you now!"* At their extreme, during these moments, events – including the appearing of a person in the room, someone's way of moving, the tone of his voice – may acquire an offensive, thing-like physiognomy, and become intruding, perforating. Borderline persons can be overly sensitive to minimal social stimuli, like for instance the other's facial expressions that pass unobserved to the majority of people. Expert clinicians know very well that borderline patients may become aware of subtle emotions that, during a session, affect the clinician and of which he himself may be unaware. Typically, the patient is not capable of integrating these "spasms" of hyper-awareness or hyper-empathy in a fluent and attuned relationship with the therapist (or with the other person in general). Instead of contributing to the development of an exchange of feelings and views between the patient and the other, they stand out as islands of immediateness, leaving no space between oneself and the other, or between oneself and one's own overwhelming insights.

These persons, therefore, live in a restricted temporal horizon and are scarcely aware of a future or a past. There are three main visible or behavioral aspects to this. First, they are frequently affected by rapid mood swings. They appear changeable, inconstant, voluble, "moody," often prey to emotional crises and attacks. Second, they appear to be trapped in present stimuli, so that, for instance, their therapeutic conversation is often a mere catalogue of recent events. Their awareness is captivated by the present moment, as if they were unable to ignore or switch off the stimuli that are coming from the environment or from their own body. These sensations may appear trivial, irrelevant, or meaningless to an external observer, but for borderline patients themselves they are abnormally important and amplified. This phenomenon cannot be explained as abnormal arousal, as is the case with anxious patients. The third feature of discontinuity of borderline personal existence analyzed by Meares (2000) includes what he calls the "traumatic system" (for details see "Narrative Self and Limit Situation" section).

Space

Dysphoria has a horizontal absorption in the sense that it attends to the world as a whole, not focusing on any particular object or situation. No particular action is dictated by dysphoric mood. On the contrary, it complicates the relation between feeling and action because it introduces doubt, hesitation, and questions. Whereas we usually organize our actions in the mode of succession, in despair movements remain stuck in the indecisiveness of juxtaposition, that is, a kind of paralysis of action and thinking, but not a static one, rather a frenzied, restless, disconcerting paralysis.

Dysphoric space is usually experienced as indifferent extension and isotropic space devoid of salience that offers no directions and no way out. We find an apparently similar phenomenon describing lived space in persons with schizophrenia. The basic difference between these two is that whereas in the schizophrenic mood lived space conveys a feeling of unreality, in borderline persons it conveys a feeling of meaninglessness.

Furthermore, when dysphoria turns into boredom, the surrounding world is "moribund" (Stanghellini and Rosfort, 2013b). One's life appears as meaningless, without scope. It is like *"still black water/as deep as forever/as cold as the sky/as still as my heart when your voice is gone/I shall freeze in hell"* (Kane, 2001: 239). In despair, space undergoes an even deeper metamorphosis. The movements remain stuck in the indecisiveness of juxtaposition. Despair in the borderline life-world is a kind of frenetic palsy. Dysphoric mood, ignited by shame, may turn into anger; then (as we shall see) space offers no protection. In despair, there is a profound alteration of lived space. Indeed, whereas we usually organize our actions in the mode of succession, in despair movements remain stuck in the indecisiveness of juxtaposition, that is, a kind of paralysis of action and thinking, but not a static one, rather a frenzied, restless, disconcerting paralysis.

Body

The emotional fragility or stable instability experienced by borderline persons while inhabiting the dysphoric life-world is caused by a raw, unmediated bodily vitality that does not accommodate to pre-reflective intentional structures or cognitive efforts. Their dysphoric mood is characterized by extreme presence of a primary, bodily force that fragments the intentional structure of human embodiment, the lived body, exposing a brutal vitality, a mere body entirely at the mercy of the basic biological values that nourish and to some extent orient human emotional life. There is little possibility for action in this kaleidoscopic universe of raw feelings. Objects become unfocused and intentional structures crumple under the intensity of this emotional pressure. Bodily reactions take dominance over bodily action, and the intimate sense of being an embodied self is eclipsed by the sense of having an intimidating body. This chaotic vitality, being devoid of intentional structure and content, desperately seeks an object, mostly a person, at which to direct its surplus of energy. This means that the dysphoric person feels the presence of a spontaneous energy without any clear direction or definite target. It is emotional energy that throws itself at the other with an overwhelming intensity. Often, this impulse takes on a sexual form which the borderline person defines as "love." The loved object is the form that the desperate vitality takes for the borderline person (Stanghellini and Rosfort, 2013b; Ractliffe and Stephan, 2014).

On one side, this power is a violent spasm that takes control of the body and destroys the embodied structure that organizes our intentional engagement with the world. It is experienced as an energy that takes the representation of oneself to pieces, reducing it to an assemblage of disordered emotions and drives. On the other side, however, it is also a power that expresses an encouraging vitality seductively in touch with invigorating sensations (Ractliffe and Stephan, 2014).

The term "dysphoria" indicates an emotional state that is hard to endure. In this case, the subject experiences a state that, literally, does not suit him. This is the meaning of the term in many psychiatric conditions, where the subject experiences a state of uncomfortableness, distress, and discomfort with respect to their own body. This is the case with so-called "gender dysphoria," in which one feels forced to inhabit a body that does not correspond to one's desired gender. Also, it is the case with premenstrual dysphoria, a body condition that hinders one's life and must be dealt with, or with neuroleptic dysphoria, a feeling of unease and discomfort related to a sense of mental and motor awkwardness, which the patient sees as an effect of the intake of neuroleptics. In short, the mood condition typical of dysphoria has to do with the perception of something that is askew – something that went wrong and hinders one's life. Indeed, in dysphoria, everything goes wrong (Stanghellini, 2016a, 2016b).

In dysphoric acute states, as in the case with dysphoric depressions, one's own body, as the source of vitality and conation, is felt as distant from oneself and out of voluntary control, lying somewhere between self and non-self – the land of otherness (Stanghellini and Rosfort, 2013b).

The sense of void is very common in borderline depression or in the micro-depressive episodes which may punctuate the borderline person's daily existence. These are the episodes during which deep feelings of depersonalization add up to the permanent lack of a stable, integral identity. Feelings of auto-, somato-, and allo-psychic depersonalization, i.e. sensations of emptiness, numbness, fragmentation, vanishing of one's own self are typically accompanied by feelings of abandonment and aloneness – all immersed in an atmosphere of *"corrosive doubt/futile despair/horror in repose"* that engenders a devastating sense of resignation: *"I can fill my space/fill my time/but nothing can fill this void in my heart"* (Kane, 2001: 219).

Precisely because dysphoria as a mood cannot be easily modulated, the only possible control is sought outside of the mind, on the surface of a body on which to inscribe one's own emotional state. Borderline self-harm is a way to find relief from the torment of inner tension. The self-inflicted lesion of the skin provides a temporary oasis of peace and relaxation. It is a way to take a rest from dysphoria (Rossi Monti and D'Agostino, 2014). This relief, however, can also be achieved by targeting the outside world, that is, by acting on the environment and transforming it even with violence.

Furthermore, the body could represent a means by which to decrease the state of tension – e.g. by self-mutilation. The cutting of the flesh represents an attempt to modulate or staunch a negative and oppressive mood condition, precipitating it in a place that has a name and is objectifiable, delimited, and so also "curable" (Rossi Monti and D'Agostino, 2014). It is as if the body can be a concrete and visible sort of drain for overwhelming emotions.

Self

According to Kernberg (1984), identity diffusion in borderline patients reflects their inability to integrate positive and negative representations of the self and the other. The result is a shifting view of the self, with sharp discontinuities, rapidly shifting roles (e.g. victim and victimizer, dominant and submissive), and a sense of inner emptiness. Wilkinson-Ryan and Westen (2000) empirically demonstrated that identity disturbance in BPD is characterized by a painful sense of incoherence, objective inconsistencies in beliefs and behaviors, over-identification with groups or roles, and, to a lesser extent, difficulties with commitment to jobs, values, and goals.

Dysphoric mood brings about a formless and immaterial sense of one's own self; a cold, black pond into which the self is drawn – the words of Sarah Kane. Yet, focusing on the vital character of dysphoria implies being able to see in the precarious sense of selfhood and identity of borderline persons a positive aspect, a less deadly feature than mere identity confusion and the manifestation of the death instinct. Dysphoric persons feel that they have the right to receive a compensation for the traumas they have suffered; they have the right to rebel against the hypocrisy of social conventions, and thus to change the world (Correale, 2007). This is the tragic horizon in which the bad mood of borderline persons is inscribed (Stanghellini, 2000a).

It should be noted that the fabric of the self (Meares, 2000) is a delicate one in the case of the dysphoric life-world. The development of a cohesive and continuous sense of self depends upon a special form of conversation: a non-linear, associative, and apparently purposeless form of dialogue, whose topic may at first glance seem banal. It is like a game, since it is apparently aimless. Or like an atmosphere, because it can be extremely difficult to answer questions about what is actually going on here or what we are really talking about. Intimacy is the basic emotion involved in this kind of conversation. Intimacy, Meares (2000) explains, is not to be equated to confession or incontinent revelation. Rather, it is the feelings in which this special kind of conversation is embedded, such as having a peculiar warmth or a form associated with a sense of well-being. Intimacy fundamentally depends upon the sharing of one's own inner experience with another.

Moreover, the integrity of the self can be damaged by traumatic experience. The kind of trauma at issue here is not sexual abuse or some form of violent behavior, but rather takes the form of an invalidating environment. An invalidating environment is one in which communication of private experiences is not met by appropriate responses. Instead of being validated, private experiences are trivialized, their expression is discouraged, and emotions (especially painful emotions) are disregarded. The kind of trauma that may jeopardize the development of a warm and intimate sense of self is the absence of recognition (Stanghellini and Rosfort, 2013b).

Other Persons

In synchrony with the drastic fluctuation of feelings, there is an instability in the appearance of other persons. In the life-world of dysphoria, others may appear as mere shadows. To use the words spoken by the patients themselves, the other is experienced as indefinite, indeterminate, indistinct, ill-defined. All these qualities that the borderline person perceives unmediated in other persons express in semi-sensorial terms the unintelligibility of the Other. The indefiniteness of the Other is the norm in borderline existence, and it worsens in acute dysphoric-depressive episodes during which the Other may become without light and opaque: fuzzy, blurred, caliginous, cloudy, foggy, gray, hazy. When the dysphoric mood turns into anger, the other changes from being opaque to being tenebrous: he is ambivalent, evasive, obscure, puzzling, un-explicit, and suspect. This paves the way to persecutory delusions (e.g.: Why don't you say explicitly you want to harm me!).

At the heart of the existence of borderline persons' drama resides the excruciating experience of the Other. The main concern of the borderline person is "to receive attention/to be seen and heard/to excite, amaze, fascinate, shock, intrigue, amuse, entertain or entice others" (Kane, 2001: 234). Also, to avoid pain and shame, repress fear, maintain self-respect; all this is needed to overcome past traumatic experiences, "to obliterate past humiliation by resumed action" (Kane, 2001: 234). The Other is indispensable for living and its absence makes the presence of the self impossible. The Other is absent when she is not totally present. Her absence, or incomplete presence, is often the reason for feelings of non-recognition and desperate loss of selfhood. The Other who does not donate her entire self is an inauthentic Other.

The Other is also the source of aching shame, since her gaze is permanently on the razor's edge between recognition and humiliation: *"Watching me, judging me … I gape in horror at the world and wonder why everyone is smiling and looking at me with secret knowledge of my aching shame/Shame shame shame./Drown in your fucking shame"* (Kane, 2001: 209).

The Other in borderline existence, first and foremost, appears as dim and fuzzy, and yet the very same Other remains a prerequisite for being a self and establishing a narrative identity (Stanghellini and Rosfort, 2013b). Yet, as we have shown in the paragraph on temporality, the borderline patient may be struck by details that remain unnoticed by the others.

The brimming intensity of the dysphoric mood demands the same intensity of the intentional correlate to its affects. Something of the desperate and frustrated energy of the dysphoric mood is transferred to the intentional structures of the interpersonal relation. The intensity of the borderline person cannot be disappointed. It is all-or-nothing. This immensely intense character of interpersonal relationships makes them highly precarious. The slightest change in the emotional atmosphere, a wrong word, a delay, and the borderline person feels attacked or humiliated, and reacts with anger.

The Life-World of Anger

Time

Anger makes a person completely identified with her momentary state of mind, unable to gain a distance from the present situation, torn by emerging impulses – i.e. bursts of anger. Therefore, wishes and impulses flare up and vanish again, driving the patients forward, but without connecting to form a long-term project (Fuchs, 2007).

In anger, borderline persons are completely absorbed by the phenomenon that agitates them. When a borderline person is angry, a relevant feature of the world (usually threatening her personal existence and the value she attaches to it) captivates her, irrupts into her field of awareness without her having decided to turn her attention to it. She becomes fixated on the object of her anger, and all her attention is captured by it.

As we have seen in describing the life-world of dysphoria, borderline persons live unhistorically, bound to a transitory present without depth (Stanghellini and Rosfort, 2013a). The borderline person is absorbed in an unmediated instantaneity (Kimura, 1992): a pure or absolute now devoid of past and future. This is also the case with anger, although with some relevant differences which we will analyze in detail in the following.

Space

Significant transformations in the experience of space may occur in the complexity of emotions that characterize the borderline existence. As we saw earlier, emotions are the "spatializing-temporalizing vortex" of the life-world.

In the life-world of anger, events are described as "wounding," "biting," "stinging." Someone's remark may be felt as "caustic," "corrosive," "dissecting"; her behavior, "pointed," "raw," "sharp" – and these, of course, are not just metaphors. Changes in lived space make it possible to experience someone's comportment as piercing; the piercing metaphors arise from alterations of lived space (Stanghellini and Rosfort, 2013a).

In general, the physiognomy of things in the life-world of borderline persons reflects the fluctuation in lived time between evanescence and urgency: things show themselves on the edge between melting and blasting. They are dissolving, liquefying (in dysphoria) as well as ardent, combusting, conflagrating (in anger): *"In a moment things around me are glowing, and a moment later reduced to ashes," "My life is as if I were walking on burning coals," "Feverish moments, during which something makes me feel fervent"* (Stanghellini and Rosfort, 2013a).

To summarize: whereas in dysphoria space is an indifferent extension devoid of salience and offers no directions and movement remains stuck in the indecisiveness of juxtaposition, in the life-world of anger space offers no protection. Space is a beeline between the angry person and the person who offended her. The offending one gains an absolute centrality around which everything else dissolves.

Body

In the grip of anger the body is impregnated by it. A numb and empty body becomes a body filled with anger. A bodily self filled with anger is a self that can finally feel itself, a strong and hard embodied self that repays the suffered insults – but at the cost of losing its humanity, and thus wrecking the fragile dialectic of selfhood and otherness constitutive of personhood. It is a self that is insensitive to the voice and the face of the other person, a self without innocence, a self that has lost its humanity. The body merely becomes a "state" of wild emotional tension bringing the person inexorably to destruction.

Self

Anger tends to preserve and maintain a precarious cohesion of the self (Pazzagli and Rossi Monti, 2000: 223), in the same way that a small child might self-inflict physical pain in order to try to keep a sense of being alive and of cohesion.

In this state anger, as we have seen, is to a certain extent a self-defining emotion. It is a self that is insensitive to the voice and the face of the other person, a self without innocence, a self that has lost the humanity endemic to personhood. Tragic is the existence which, in pursuing a plan, acts in such a way that it brings the same plan inexorably to destruction. This is the case for the borderline person's anger, which seems to be situated at the point where an intention swings into its opposite: fragile doubts about oneself and the other into incorrigible convictions, moral indignation into the shame of aggression, the fire of love into the stake of intolerance (Stanghellini, 2000a).

This is indeed the place of emotions like shame and humiliation that pave the way to the outburst of anger. The life-world of shame to a certain extent parallels that of anger (as the life-world of boredom matches the one of dysphoria). More precisely, we can say that the experience of shame precedes the experience of anger. I feel seen by another person whose piercing gaze nails me to a part of myself that makes me feel humiliated. I feel my body deprived of any protection and at the same time dirtied. Lived time comes to a fixation in an instant that grows to infinity. Yet shame, as compared to dysphoria, is a feeling that restores a sense of self-identity and self-recognition, although confined to a part of one's self. The effect of shame is that it reduces the nebula of feelings conveyed by dysphoria to one single feature: my stain. Reducing my identity to my defect, it restores a primitive sense of selfhood.

Anger often comes as a reaction to shame and humiliation, which makes the person lose her opportunity to contact and recognize that part of oneself that the other's gaze has revealed. When shame turns into anger we forget that we must feel shame because of our being a continuous movement and a transition in which the gaze of the other serves to acknowledge our limitations and to come to terms with our *guiltless guilt*.

Anger tends to preserve and maintain a precarious cohesion of the self (Pazzagli and Rossi Monti, 2000: 223), in the sense that venting one's anger is a way of feeling alive and of affirming one's right to exist as the unique person that one is. In anger episodes, the vague and confused sense of values and norms that characterizes borderline existence is suddenly replaced by a crystal clear, although elementary normative, universe in which it is painfully obvious to the borderline person who is "good" (oneself) and who is "bad" (the other). This sudden feeling of infallible rightness helps the borderline person to find his or her lost identity in a world that momentarily regains its structure and meaning.

Other Persons

First of all, anger is the means through which the borderline patient reacts to every minimal break in empathy: anger emerges when the patient feels that the other will not perform the function he desperately needs. In fact, anger makes the object clearly visible, strongly characterized and standing out very distinctively. It allows the BPD patient to switch from the state of vagueness typical of dysphoric mood (where the object is blurred, nebulous, and ambiguous) to a condition in which the object is crisp and clear. In this sense, anger has a "centripetal" role, coagulating the emotional dispersion by identifying each time an object/ interlocutor (Rossi Monti and D'Agostino, 2014). Furthermore, anger defends from the pain of separation and loss: a mind kept busy by angry fantasies somehow is still clinging to what it has lost (Rossi Monti and D'Agostino, 2014). In the light of anger, which dissipates the hazy atmosphere of dysphoria, the other suddenly comes into focus as a persecutor. The gaze of the other mercilessly lays bare the patient's inner insufficiency and thus makes her feel humiliated. So, the sense of identity established by anger is highly unstable due to the fact that the cohesion brought about by anger is constantly threatened by the instability brought about by humiliation. Moreover, feelings of abandonment, or lack of attention, acceptance, help, protection, reciprocity, support – or in short, lack of recognition – are typical in the borderline traumatic existence. The borderline person looks primarily in the direction of the other. It is the other who is guilty, since he or she acted out of voluntary intention. These feelings may kindle acute emotional states characterized by anger, resentment, and indignation. The self–other relationship may take the form of a transitory persecutory delusion (Stanghellini and Rosfort, 2013c).

Narrative Self and Limit Situation

As we saw above, the persons with BPD lack "object constancy" in the sense of being able to retain a positive image of significant others in spite of temporary separation or rejection. The result is what Fuchs (2007) has called a fragmentation of the narrative self: a shifting view of oneself, with sharp discontinuities, rapidly changing representations of oneself and others, and an underlying feeling of inner emptiness. There is no sense of continuity over time and across situations, no concept of self-development that could be projected into the future, but only an endless repetition of the same emotional states, creating a peculiar a-temporal mode of existing. The patients often rapidly change their goals, jobs, and friends as well as their convictions and values; they are unable to commit themselves to a set of self-defining values, enduring relationships, and long-term aspirations (Westen and Cohen, 1993).

The temporal fragmentation of the self, Fuchs argues, avoids the necessity of tolerating the threatening ambiguity and uncertainty of interpersonal relationships. The price, however, consists in a chronic feeling of inner emptiness caused by the inability to integrate past and future into the present and, thus, to establish a coherent sense of identity. Being ruled only by their momentary emotions and impulses, i.e. first-order desires, borderline persons lack an essential feature of being a person, namely the capacity of self-conducing/directing. Thus, apparently, the mode of existence of borderline persons is not just a defense in a strict sense, but a kind of necessity entailed by these persons' lack of the strength to establish a coherent personal identity through a labor of temporal integration.

Temporal integration and narrative identity are closely intertwined. Narrative identity implies a meaningful coherence of the personal past, present, and future. This meaningful coherence is not already there. Rather, it is the product of an enduring labor striving to make one's life coherent and to fill it with meaningful behavior. Narrative identity is different from mere constancy or sameness, since it is a temporal relation to oneself – in view of the continuing task of becoming the person that one is – by remaining faithful to one's commitments, promises, and responsibilities in front of other people ("keeping one's word," Ricoeur, 1992: 118). It also requires the capacity of self-determination by forming durable second-order volitions, at the price, if necessary, of repression or neurosis. In the existence of borderline persons we find no consistent endeavor to do this. They lack the capacity to form enduring second-order volitions, in the light of which present impulses could be evaluated and selected.

An essential feature of the borderline persons' life-world is that typically these persons are not able to distance themselves from present events. As space offers little or no protection from piercing objects, neither does time protect from wounding memories. This is the key to understanding the traumatic existence of borderline persons. The present moment irrupts without mediation into the existence of borderline persons. Borderline persons are not able to liberate themselves from what they are thinking, experiencing, or suffering right now. The incapacity to distance oneself from an event, to take a stance in front of it, to integrate it into a narrative sequence and by doing so to give a personal meaning to it, are defining characteristics of trauma. A trauma is an event that the person is not able to appropriate, i.e. to integrate into her narrative identity. Our existence is moved forward by what happens in our life. Events happen to us as a part of involuntary otherness involved in a human life, and we appropriate these events, or we define ourselves in opposition to these events; but no matter how we relate ourselves to the events of our life, our sheer relation, our position-taking, instills personal meaning in them, and by this activity we affirm our selfhood. This dialectic of otherness and selfhood is at the heart of the construction of our narrative identity. If an event loses this capacity to "move," the dialectic of identity shatters because the person is not able to integrate this event into the historicity of his or her existence. The event becomes a traumatic event, it becomes pathogenic. An event is traumatic when it does not kindle the dialectic of narrative identity – rather, it arrests the historicity of existence (Stanghellini and Rossi Monti, 2009a, 2009b).

Borderline persons live out a traumatic existence because they are not able to *think otherwise*. They cannot articulate the present with their past – they cannot view their present experience as the product of past ones. Also, they are incapable of distancing themselves from the present experience and by doing so to take a different stance towards it, that is, to view their present from a different angle (Stanghellini and Rosfort, 2013a).

The frequency of traumatic experiences is significantly higher in BPD than in other personality disorders or in depression. However, BPD can develop without any trauma history (Paris, 1994), and trauma is a risk factor for many other mental disorders (Paris, 2000). Moreover, around 80 percent of people exposed to early trauma do not develop mental disorders (Mullen and Fergusson, 1999). The idea that BPD is rooted in early trauma is probably overrated and may lead to wrong interpretations. Clinicians should not automatically assume that present traumatic experiences are re-enactments of early traumatic experiences. Correale (2007) advises clinicians to transfer the focus of attention during therapy sessions from the search for early psychological adversities to the *daily traumas* suffered by these patients. This is not to deny the importance of child abuse or neglect in the pathogenesis of this condition. Rather, it is a way to meet the patients' need to recount their traumatic existence, and to enhance the patients' capacity to describe their experiences and reflect upon them by placing them in time and history. This, of course, will also improve the clinician's understanding of what is actually going on in the patient's life-world. We suggests focusing on what we call "traumatic sequence," performing with the patient a kind of slow motion recollection of one of the daily traumatic events that constellate her existence. According to Correale (2007), the clinician should ask the patient *to explicate* her own experience, to give further details about the traumatic sequence and the emotions involved in it. *Explication* here means bringing out the raw feelings of the patient's experiences and the personal meanings that the patient attributes to them. It is an accurate unfolding of subjective experiences and the organization of these experiences according to a meaningful pattern immanent to the experiences themselves; the interpretation or the explanation of these experiences according to a model that is not immanent in the clinical material itself may come as a later step (Stanghellini and Rossi Monti, 2009a).

Typically, the traumatic sequence includes four steps:

(1) As we have seen, the relationships of borderline persons are often traumatic. The borderline person is not capable of autonomy in the sense of establishing a coherent enough representation of herself and remaining faithful to it, and thus takes to an extreme the value of spontaneity. She conceives of partnerships as the encounter between two spontaneities, not regulated by any sort of internal or external *nomos* (Stanghellini and Rosfort, 2013a, 2013b). Furthermore, the borderline person requires

the other to be present and loyal, and capable of recognition, that is, a source of validation. In addition, presence, loyalty, and recognition must be accompanied by the other's spontaneity, being free from social conventions and acting according to the vital impulses of the present moment.

(2) A phase of emotional dissonance and cognitive indecision. The traumatic sequence typically starts with an unexpected event of disappointment and disillusion. The other does something (or omits to do something) and thereby hurts the borderline person's sensibility. Indeed, the borderline person is incapable of renouncing her/his sensibility because she/he cannot perceive the other as a social role, that is, as an external representative of identity. Usually, in this phase, the borderline persons are overwhelmed by a quasi-ineffable variety of bad moods, including dysphoria, anxiety, and despair, characterized on the cognitive level by a state of dissonance and indecision. This is an initial manifestation of what is sometimes called the borderline patient's deficit of reflective function (Fonagy and Target, 1997). We prefer to talk of her difficulty in situating her emotions. To situate one's emotions means to recognize and relate them to the present situation, to understand them as one's own personal way of being attuned to that given situation; and eventually to grasp the connection between one's emotions, the present situation in which they are elicited, and one's life-history as the background from which they arise. Borderline persons fail to see in their emotional reactions the involuntary manifestation of otherness, that is, the re-enactment of one's past and the manifestation of one's character. Thus, they fail to engage in a proper "hermeneutics of the I am" (Stanghellini and Rosfort, 2013a).

(3) Emotional dissonance is prodromal to a phase of despair. It concerns a kind of frenzied paralysis of action and thinking. Despair may be the ingress into dissociation, which is often considered a desperate defense or adaptation to traumatic experiences. In the state of dissociation there is a collapse of the capacity of mentalization. Dissociation may imply amnesia, and therefore this phase may be absent in the patient's spontaneous recollection of the traumatic sequence.

(4). The last step of the traumatic sequence is a mechanical, routine interpretation of the traumatic event. The borderline person typically assumes one of the following stereotyped roles: victim, perpetrator, bystander (see for details the section on "Guidelines for Interviewing Persons with BPD").

Limit situations for the borderline person always originate in the context of traumatic self–other relationships. The relationships of borderline persons are often traumatic. The reasons for this, as we have tried to explain, are of two primary kinds. First, there is a difficulty in establishing an image or representation of one's partner coherent over time, since the dysphoria–anger complex entails an oscillation between an opaque (fuzzy, blurred, hazy) image of the other, and an image of the other as tenebrous (ambivalent, evasive, obscure, puzzling, suspect). Second, the values at play in the interpersonal world of borderline persons are not only difficult to attain, but in conflict with one another. The borderline person needs the other to be a source of recognition and validation. He or she requires the other to be present, reliable and loyal over time, but at the same time he or she wants the other to be spontaneous and authentic "right now."

Meares (2000) pinpoints an essential feature of the fabric of the human self that is missing in the life-story of borderline persons. This is the issue of the other's recognition, which is missing in the circumstances that Meares calls the "invalidating trauma." Our concern for the other originates in a lack in our own existence that generates a need for a dialogical coexistence with the other. We do not need the other merely as a means to satisfy our own desires. This need for others drastically affects the value I attach to myself. When the other person addresses me "in the second person, I feel I am implicated in the first person" (Ricoeur, 1992: 193). The other person is fundamental to my own sense of being a self, to my self-esteem, and to my identity, because the world is a shared world whose meaning is, for the major part, constituted by the coexistence of different persons. My identity as a person depends on the other's recognition of my being so. The unity and coherence of my various actions with respect to the idea of myself as an individual person is deeply influenced by the reception of these actions by other persons – and this process is embedded in a special kind of intimate conversation during which I recognize the other as a oneself and the oneself as an other (Ricoeur, 1992: 194). Meares's argument on this point is very close to the importance Kimura (1992) attributes to the interpersonal *aïda* in the constitution of the self, but compared to Kimura he adds a very important element. He sets the fabric of the self in an emotional atmosphere, since to him intimacy is a prerequisite for a mature self to develop, i.e. a self at ease in dialoguing with itself (Stanghellini and Rosfort, 2013a). Of course, this is also an extremely relevant point with respect to the issue of care. As we shall see in the next section, the presence of the other (and of intimacy) as a companion for my inner conversations is a prerequisite for the temporal continuity of my narrative identity.

Values in Persons with BPD

BPD patients tend to be hyper-reactive to environmental stimuli. As we saw in the section on their life-worlds, the borderline existence is characterized by unpleasant and often very painful emotions that can become destructive generally or self-destructive in desperate attempts to get out of this emotional state. This can be seen as the results from the cyclical emotional oscillation between hope for stability and disappointment in its unattainability. A dependent-anaclitic depression may arise from these contrasting needs and desires, whose typical features are a mixture of anger, aloneness, and inner emptiness. The tendency to be immersed in the here-and-now (*intra festum*) exacerbates the sense of isolation, causing profound irritation, mute frustration, and, consequently, anger.

The desperate vitality inherent in dysphoria engenders an intense need to satisfy the affective, biological values brought about by vigorous feelings of being alive. These values run counter to and often clash with the ethical norms and social rules that structure the world in which we all live, provoking a frustrated sense of worthlessness and inanity. The emotional intensity does not allow the person to distance themselves from what they feel here and now, and therefore they are not able to understand their feelings in the light of the values that constitute their own life-world. They live under the spell of what we may call a *frustrated normativity* (Stanghellini and Rosfort, 2013a, 2013b). The norms by which the borderline person is driven are not the ethical norms or social conventions that structure and organize our interpersonal world. Rather, borderline persons refuse such conditions, thus entering into collision with what they consider the hypocrisy and the inauthenticity of the pallid emotions by which other persons live.

The borderline person's normativity is an emotional normativity constituted by the intensity of affective values which are nevertheless constantly frustrated by the ethical norms and the social rules and conventions that structure our interpersonal world. The borderline person cannot – or will not – let his bouts of energy be restricted by or conformed to the needs of other people, ethical norms, or social conventions, all of which he considers inauthentic and therefore as an unwarranted challenge to his truly natural being, his spontaneity.

This kind of emotionally frustrated normativity can be the initial cause of borderline depression. It is the presence of a vitality that merely strives to affirm its own emotional intensity, to satisfy its own rudimentary feelings of being alive and the anonymous values revealed and engendered by these feelings, without any regard for the ethical or social norms that govern the world in which the borderline person desperately tries to live. Feelings and values are the same for the borderline person. They can only feel the meaning of values. Norms are inauthentic because they disregard the intimate feelings of the person whose behavior they are meant to inform and orient. The incapacity to distance oneself from one's own feelings means that the borderline person is not capable of appropriating those very feelings in the light of the norms that are part of being a person in a world shared with other persons. She is condemned to simply live the intense but disrupted life of her feelings. The norms, ethical as well as social, that allow us to distance ourselves from our feelings and needs in the light of our care for living "a good life" with other people are somehow undermined by the intensity of the borderline feelings. Norms and conventions are merely viewed as annoying attempts to drain the vitality that sustains the borderline world. The normative frustration experienced by borderline persons continuously generates desperate attempts to maintain their vitality in the face of what they consider to be the encumbering strictures and platitudes of everyday life. In general, vitality and desire in borderline persons are closely related to a kind of enjoyment characterized by its impossibility in essence. Yet borderline persons experience this primordial enjoyment as *forbidden* (and as such as inviting transgression) rather than as simply *impossible* (Mooij, 2012: 190).

The values that are at play in the interpersonal world of borderline persons are directed to achieve apparently standard (but in fact unattainable) goals like *"to belong/to be accepted/ to draw close and enjoyably reciprocate with another/to converse in a friendly manner, to tell stories, exchange sentiments, ideas, secrets/to communicate, to converse/to laugh and make jokes"* (Kane, 2001: 234–235). These goals are felt by borderline persons as standard, basic aspirations of what, with Meares (2000), we may call intimacy, but these aspirations are often unrealistic and almost unattainable.

Not only do the borderline person's values clash with the norms and conventions that rule our interpersonal world. The values at play in the interpersonal world of borderline persons are not only difficult to attain, but in conflict with one another. More intimate, personal values are also entailed in the borderline person's ideal of being with others. The borderline person requires the other to be present and loyal, and capable of recognition, that is, a source of validation. In addition, presence, loyalty, and recognition must be accompanied by the other's spontaneity, being free from social conventions and acting according to the vital impulses of the present moment. Furthermore, as we have seen, the borderline person is not capable of autonomy in the sense of establishing a coherent enough representation of herself and remaining faithful to it, and thus takes to an extreme the value of spontaneity. They conceive of partnerships as the encounter between two spontaneities, not regulated by any sort of internal or external *nomos*: *"to be free from social restrictions/to resist coercion and constriction/to be independent and act according to desire/to defy convention"* (Kane, 2001: 234).

Love, Authenticity, and the Desperate Need for Recognition

As we have described in the section concerning other persons in the borderline life-world, in the borderline existence, the other is seen as: (1) dim and fuzzy; (2) a source of recognition; (3) an abandoning other who does not donate her entire self.

Borderline persons live in the glorification of an authentic encounter with the Other (Stanghellini, 2016a). Authenticity here means the striving for an immediate and mystic fusion with the Other. Obviously, on this basis the encounter can only fail.

The borderline person postulates, in fact, as essential to life what is more alien and inaccessible to it, what in life itself is unstable and fleeting par excellence: the immediate encounter with the Other, the encounter between two desires. The imperatives shouted at the other are the following: "Spontaneously fulfill my desire with your own desire!" and "Stay here! Do not abandon me! Keep on burning with an inexhaustible desire!"

Need for recognition and fear of abandonment force the borderline person to aspire – constantly and insatiably – to a sort of emotional osmosis with the Other. The Other is needed as a source of recognition. The absence of the Other makes the presence of the self impossible. The Other's absence, or incomplete presence, is often the reason for feelings of un-recognition and desperate loss of selfhood. The absent Other, or the Other who does not donate his entire self, is an abandoning Other and an inauthentic Other.

We know how an encounter based on these needs (immediacy and authenticity) is unrealistic and almost unattainable. Furthermore, the borderline's desire conceals the difference between oneself and the Other, and between one's desire for love and love in its actuality. In short: between an idealized form of love and the actual relationship with the other person. What the borderline person idealizes is not the Other, but Love itself.

Quoting Roland Barthes (2001: 22):

> *Against and in spite of everything, the subject affirms love as value*: Despite the difficulties of my story, despite discomforts, doubts, despairs, despite impulses to be done with it, *I unceasingly affirm love, within myself, as a value.* Though I listen to all the arguments which the most divergent systems employ to demystify, to limit, to erase, in short to depreciate love, I persist: "I know, I know, but all the same . . ." I refer the devaluations of love to a kind of obscurantist ethic, to a let's-pretend realism, against which I erect the realism of value: I counter whatever "doesn't work" in love with the affirmation of what is worthwhile. This stubbornness is love's protest: for all the wealth of "good reasons" for loving differently, loving better, loving without being in love, etc., a stubborn voice is raised which lasts a little longer: the voice of the Intractable lover.

What the borderline person considers to be her most non-renounceable value is indeed her innermost symptom. The borderline existence is a dangerous shelter that meets its defeat because it postulates as non-renounceable in life what is more alien and inaccessible to it, what in life itself is unstable and fleeting par excellence: the immediate encounter with the Other, the encounter between two desires.

Guidelines for Interviewing Persons with BPD: Responsibility without Blame

The therapeutic interview with borderline persons is a very difficult task because they easily feel blamed for their deeds. Shame is the emotion elicited by the gaze of another person that reveals a feature of myself that makes me feel inadequate. When I feel ashamed, I feel that the other's piercing gaze nails me to my *stain* and that, for the other, I am nothing but that stain.

This painful feeling, instead of helping BPD patients to focus on their actions and eventually acknowledge their responsibility, usually kindles an intense emotional reaction that makes them feel the victim of an unjust accusation. Experiencing shame re-enacts a victim–perpetrator self-with-other relational scheme. This enactment is not only extremely painful, but also impedes the BPD patient to get an insight into the meaning of her feeling of shame, that is, what shame can reveal about her existence.

To avoid this, the interviewer must be aware of the complex nature of the feeling of shame as the emotion that reveals the "claire-obscure" of human existence (Scheler, 1928/2012). The dark and astonishing feeling of shame arises from the experience of the clash between what ideally "ought to be" and what, in fact, is: an imbalance and disharmony in man between the sense and the claim of spiritual values and embodied or organic needs. Shame arises from the contiguity between higher levels of ethical conscience and lower drive-awareness.

Shame as "guiltless guilt" also reveals the fold of voluntary and involuntary, activity and passivity, and, more in general, responsibility and non-responsibility in human existence. Agency and responsibility reveal a fold in human existence. There are several reasons for this:

(1) They cannot be easily disentangled on the ontological level. To be human is to be at odds with agency, that is, with the involuntary dimension of our being which does not fully separate from the involuntary.

(2) Responsibility reveals a fold in human existence since it is at the same time a presupposition and a task. It is a presupposition since society expects a person to feel responsible for her deeds. It is a task since responsibility is not a priori in human existence; rather it is an achievement to be obtained through education.

(3) The fold that unites responsibility and non-responsibility cannot easily unfold on the ethical level. To be human is at the same time to be aware that we cannot fully control the involuntary dimension of our existence, and that we are held responsible for it.

Let it be said that between voluntary and involuntary, between responsibility and non-responsibility, there is a sort of continuity. In this fold, there is a zone of undecidability. This fold is primarily felt and experienced as an obscure and perturbing entanglement of selfhood and otherness. The unfolding, before unfolding the pleat, shows the fold where the voluntary and the involuntary are continuous with each other. Explication reveals *complication* (Stanghellini, 2016a, 2016b).

The seeing of this zone of undecidability generates, depending on position-taking, feelings of guilt or feelings of alienation, or the moral emotions of shame which exactly reveal that it is not possible to decide objectively whether one's action is voluntarily or involuntarily generated. Position-taking decides whether I'm responsible or not. Whether I see myself as guilty or alienated from the source of my actions depends on the side of the fold that is visible from my perspective. To restore a full sense of responsibility, that is, to overcome alienation or guilt, I need to acknowledge the presence of the fold, to recognize it as a necessity, to move around the fold and take a different perspective on it, and finally to achieve a panoramic view on the fold. Therefore, unfolding is an act that opens up possibilities – developments and evolution – for the future. Unfolding is a practice that restores a sense of agency, and with it a sense of responsibility. The choice to unfold is an ethical choice, an act of care, a choice that has practical consequences, not a mere act of knowledge.

The borderline condition is a paradigmatic case study of the entanglement of the voluntary and the involuntary, and of the way we may help patients deal with their fold. In discovering otherness in themselves, borderline persons discover in themselves an amorphous and untamed presence. This presence is felt as a spring of disordered vitality that is a menace to autonomy in the sense of self-organization. Otherness is an impossibility for borderline persons. It is both a threat to the Self and the source of vitality, the vital force that they cannot renounce. Thus, it is impossible both to appropriate one's otherness and to distance oneself from it.

Shame and guilt, the voluntary and the involuntary, fate and necessity are the folds in which the borderline person is involved. Borderline persons may see this fold from three different angles – victim, perpetrator, bystander – and typically oscillate between these perspectives.

In particular:

(1) *Victim.* This is typical in the traumatic situation. One may identify with the role of the *victim*, and in this case feel passively involved and totally without responsibility for what happens. If I am the victim, then the other is the perpetrator. The borderline person looks primarily in the direction of the Other. It is the Other who is guilty, since he or she acted out of voluntary intention. From this Self–Other relationship can emerge emotional states characterized by anger, resentment, and indignation until they may take the form of a transitory persecutory delusion. Usually, the persecutor is a significant Other. This makes the persecutory delusions of borderline persons radically different from paranoid delusions in persons with schizophrenia, which typically involve anonymous others. Furthermore, borderline persons are more vulnerable to developing feelings of shame. Finally, a mixture of anger plus shame may trigger persecutory delusions in borderline persons, and especially delusions of reference, which typically arise in the type of borderline persons who are particularly vulnerable to narcissistic rage associated with feelings of humiliation.

(2) *Perpetrator.* The borderline person may admit she misbehaved. Nonetheless, the person thinks that she or he cannot be held entirely responsible. It was for her a sort of reflex, an automatic response she simply could not control: "I am bad, but I am not guilty because it's not my fault." Indeed, borderline persons seldom develop feelings of guilt or guilt delusions as melancholic persons do. The cause of one's actions is placed neither on a flesh-and-blood Other (one's partner, the therapist, or a friend) nor on an anonymous, generalized Other, nor a mechanism (as is the case with schizophrenic paranoid delusions of alien control). Rather, one may experience the influx in one's life of an uncontrollable destructive force that comes from within. Borderline persons are the witnesses of an ultimate truth: they feel the alienating power of the involuntary, that is, of the otherness that is constitutive of our personhood.

(3) *Bystander.* Here, the borderline person is a merely passive spectator of ineluctable and unpredictable events. One feels one cannot decide, control, or change the course of one's life: "It always goes like this. This happened again. I can do nothing to avoid it." One feels prone to develop feelings of impotence and helplessness, and to conceive of life as nonsensical. Oppressed with tedium, one's mind becomes a mirror that reflects the ineluctability of the world and one's own powerlessness, that is, the futility of existence. The world and life itself simply is; it just happens. Tedium may be interrupted by cynical, sarcastic, or auto-sarcastic remarks. In this case, neither is

the Other construed as a perpetrator nor is the Self felt as dominated by otherness. The responsibility is on sheer life itself, on its inescapable as well as unpredictable nature. Existence is a tragic existence. One feels near to one's own destiny, so much that one can see it, touch it, nearly manipulate it, and maybe avoid it. Nonetheless, one can merely watch oneself thrown into this without any brakes. The nightmare is the most common paradigm of the tragic. In every nightmare there is always a moment in which powerlessly I see myself being hurled into the jaws of the destructive power from which I was trying to escape. Borderline persons construe themselves as the bystanders of their tragic destiny. The ability to make decisions and to change their own life is absent. People with BPD are not simply unable and irresolute with life events, but they are as knocked out, stunned, impotent, and bored. As we said in the first section of this chapter, an emotional state that characterizes the borderline existence is the boredom that reflects the ineluctability of the world and one's own powerlessness, that is, the futility of existence. Barthes's example summarizes this position: "I have withdrawn from all finality, I live according to chance (as is evidenced by the fact that the figures of my discourse occur to me like so many dice casts). Flouted in my enterprise (as it happens), I emerge from it neither victor nor vanquished: I am tragic. (Someone tells me: this kind of love is not viable. But how can you evaluate viability? Why is the viable a Good Thing? Why is it better to last than to burn?)" (Barthes, 2001: 23).

Table 13.2 The life-world of borderline persons

	Experiences	
Existential	**Dysphoria**	**Anger**
Time	Monotonousness; instantaneousness; pure presentification	Impulses flare up and vanish again Complete absorption by the phenomenon that agitates them
Space	Indifferent extension; isotropic space devoid of salience	Absolute centrality of the offending one Everything else dissolves
Body	Raw, unmediated bodily vitality Bodily force that fragments the structure of human embodiment Desperate vitality.	Filled with anger the bodily self can feel itself
Other	Indefinite, indeterminate, indistinct, ill-defined	The other suddenly comes into focus as a persecutor
Self	Formless and immaterial	Precarious cohesion of the self I (borderline patient) am good and you (the other) is bad
Values:	Authenticity Immediacy Need for recognition	
Emotions	Boredom Shame Guilt	

The fold of voluntary and involuntary, selfhood and otherness is the cypher of human existence. Of this zone of undecidability, potentially tragic and despairing, the borderline person is nothing but the extreme expression. Thus the patient is held responsible, but not blameworthy for his deeds, as we as human beings are responsible but not to be blamed for our vulnerable condition (Stanghellini, 2016a, 2016b).

In a therapeutic context, the borderline person feels blamed if the therapist advocates their responsibility in the course of actions in which they are involved. The therapist should therefore adopt a stance that we could call after Hanna Pickard (2013), responsibility without blame. It consists in holding the patient responsible and accountable for harm or wrongdoing, including self-harm, without blaming him for it. The clinician's attitude should reflect the recognition of the complex equilibrium between the voluntary and involuntary dimensions in human action, and take seriously the patient's tragic awareness of this. The awareness of the fold that holds together the voluntary and the involuntary must be kept in mind to acknowledge with the patient that his degree of responsibility is reduced, yet that he could not have behaved in that given way, so he is at least partly responsible for his deeds. Responsibility is essential to help the patient restore a sense of self-cohesion and agency.

It is essential to maintain responsibility and to avoid blame in order to enable the patient to re-establish a dialogue with himself, that is, with the chiasm of voluntary and involuntary, selfhood and otherness that constitutes a human person. Patients cannot even begin to embark on this dialogue if they and those who work with them do not believe it is *in their power to do so* – that is, in their capacity for agency. This is why *responsibility* is essential for engagement and effective treatment, especially for patients with personality disorders. This can include encouraging them to see the fold of the voluntary and the involuntary from different and multiple perspectives. Table 13.2 summarizes the life-world of borderline persons.

The Life-World of Persons with Schizophrenia

Schizophrenia is a complex psychopathological condition that defies simple description. Mainstream descriptive psychopathology chiefly focuses on signs and symptoms like delusions, hallucinations, and so-called "negative symptoms" that are supposed to be relevant for diagnosis. A consequence of this tunnel vision is that much of the life-world of persons with schizophrenia remains out of view. In this chapter, we will first offer an overview of the emotional qualities of the schizophrenic form of life. Then we will characterize the schizophrenic phenotype as a whole illustrating the basic structures of the life-world within which each single abnormal experience is situated, including time, space, body, self and others, and their modifications. In the concluding part of this chapter we will turn to the description of the value-structure of persons with schizophrenia.

Temperament and Mood in Persons with Schizophrenia

The schizophrenic person's positive and negative symptoms are nothing but a superstructure, the ossification of anomalies in their emotional life. Ernst Kretschmer (1921/1961) was the first to discover the key to understanding the complexity of the emotional temperament of schizoid and schizophrenic persons. He argued that they have a surface and a depth. "Cuttingly brutal, dull and sulky, bitingly sarcastic, or timidly retiring, like a mollusk without a shell – that is the surface" (Kretschmer, 1921/1961: 146). What lurks within this dark façade? "Many schizoid folk are like Roman houses and villas, which have closed their shutters before the rays of the burning sun; perhaps in the subdued interior life, there are festivities" (Kretschmer, 1921/1961: 146).

Apparently, schizoid persons according to their emotional basic tonality can be distributed in three main groups:

(i) the humorless, serious, quiet, reserved, eccentric, unsociable type;
(ii) the timid, shy, excitable, nervous, sensitive type;
(iii) the silent, dull-witted, indifferent type.

Yet, what we can easily realize is that all these elements are inextricably mixed up with one another. The schizoid temperament lies between the extremes of excitability and dullness, indolence and anxiety and animosity. "[C]rampedness and lameness in one picture" (Kretschmer, 1921/1961: 158). These persons are over-sensitive and cold at the same time, although in quite different relational mixtures. This mixture of hyper-aesthetic and anaesthetic elements is called by Kretschmer the "psycho-aesthetic proportion" and is the core of the emotional paradox that characterizes schizophrenic spectrum disorders (Sass, 2004). Flat affect coexists with hypersensitivity to emotional stimuli. Hyper-aesthetic patients may look for protection in certain cold, or aristocratic, or manneristic attitudes. In order to understand the social eccentric behavior of people affected by schizophrenia, their eclectic sociability spanning from wax-like malleability to stubborn refusal of social norms, one needs to bring into focus the paradoxical nature of their emotional life.

A second, but not less important aspect of schizophrenic emotionality is the kind of mood that accompanies the prodromal stages of schizophrenia and culminates in the beginning of schizophrenia (see Berrios, 1996: 115–125). Patients "feel uncanny [*unheimlich*] ... Everything gets a new meaning. The environment is somehow different" (Jaspers, 1997: 98). The contents of experience may remain unchanged in themselves and yet everything appears in the light of a subtle, all penetrating, uncertain, and uncanny atmosphere. Patients feel that "they have lost grip on things" (Jaspers, 1997: 98). This is clearly an abnormal kind of mood characterized by the absence of an intentional object (see Chapter 8). This mood is also called *trema* (Conrad, 1966). It is a paradoxical mixture of anguish, hope, despair, and suspicion whereby reality becomes suspended between meaninglessness and the imminent revelation of a new meaningfulness. It characterizes the prodromal, pre-delusional stages of schizophrenia where everything feels strange, ominous, uncannily transformed; reality has undergone some inexplicable, ineffable, ungraspable change. The world is pervaded by a kind of latent meaningfulness: it has lost its habitual familiarity, and has not yet acquired a new kind of significance. Understanding reality and acting upon it has the character of achievement for patients. The condition of perennial beginners in this disorder is the *eidos* of what is accounted by phenomenological psychopathology as the matrix of the early stages of schizophrenia as well as its sub-apophanic forms.

During *trema* are clearly suspended two fundamental functions of emotion: engagement and enactment. A minimization of the relative intensity of emotions, i.e. a de-intensifying of emotional attachments and a decrease of the cathexis value of my desires, implies that one's "urgency of life" – the root of all drives, needs, and vital attention – is switched off. This kind of emotional state entails a free-floating state of consciousness (Scheler, 1973). If the urgency of life (*Lebensdrang*) is switched off, the ready-to-hand meanings of things in the world will fade away too. This implies a loss of practical references to the world – things in the world lose their practical meanings. Things in the world will not directly and immediately relate to my body as existentially relative utensils. They become non-utilizable, and as such meaningless. Things in the world appear as deprived of meanings. They are not *pragmata*, that is, equipment, something in-order-to. This brings about a radical transformation of the lived world whose main features are the abandonment of all existentially relative handles on things and a metamorphosis of lived space that grows homogeneous, isotropic, that is, devoid of any salience or point of orientation.

The suspension of my own life's urge or subjective will will preclude all interactions not only between myself and things in the world, but also all interactions between things themselves. The result of this is a perfectly adynamic world – nothing has an effect on anything else. As with causality, space and time too will undergo a deep metamorphosis. All categories we use to organize our perception of the world will vanish, including the inside/outside distinction. This radical transformation of the self–world (or body–things) relationship will enact an "essentialization" of the world in the way it is experienced, through which the world itself is transformed into an *idea*. Things will lose their incarnated givenness and be reduced to the realm of mere disembodied representations. In such a way, the world will become a perfectly ghostly world.

The third emotional dimension of schizophrenia entails a crisis of attunement. We will describe it in detail in the paragraph dedicated to the crisis of intersubjectivity. Without this capacity for emotional resonance others and the social world in general will appear mechanical and incomprehensible. The human world appears distant; there is a shutdown of the person's sense of cohesion with other human beings, and harrowing feelings of detachment from other persons, mankind, and social situations. The ability to directly contact and intuitively decipher the behavior of others and social situations is impaired. This feeling of being extraneous to the social world and of lacking an implicit, spontaneous, and emotional basis for sociality is sometimes accompanied by a numinous feeling of unity with others.

Let us now turn to the analysis of the main dimensions of the life-world that persons with schizophrenia live in.

Lived Time

Temporality constitutes the bedrock of any experience and its integrity is fundamental for the sense of coherence and continuity of selfhood and personal identity as well as for the identity through time of an object of perception. Therefore, the disintegration of time consciousness has serious psychopathological consequences for the way one experiences the phenomenal world and relates to oneself, and this is obvious in schizophrenia.

Experienced time in persons with schizophrenia is altered in its flow, being experienced as frozen, immobilized, without "élan vital" (Minkowski, 1933/1970). The loss of vital contact signifies a morbid change in the temporo-spatial structure of experiencing, particularly in the diminishment and modification of temporal-dynamic aspects and a corresponding predominance of spatial-static factors. Minkowski documented that time experience in persons with schizophrenia is characterized by the loss of immediate attunement with the present situation and they are also affected by the spatialization of time experience: time is felt as divided in juxtaposed elements that the schizophrenic person doesn't weld and gather. Moreover, persons with schizophrenia are also described as living in an elusive, eternal, and pregnant "now," that Kimura (1992) called the *ante festum*, in which what is most important is always about to happen. In a series of essays, Kimura attempts to define the kind of temporalization that characterizes persons with schizophrenia. The gist of his thesis is the following: the autonomization of the anticipating moment, disconnected from its normal interrelation with the retentional one, is the essential character of schizophrenic temporality. He calls this existential mode typical for persons with schizophrenia *ante festum* temporality. Although Kimura's analyses are not about the early stages of schizophrenia, his in-depth investigation of the changes of temporality in schizophrenic existence is nonetheless pertinent to the issue at hand. Quoting von Weizsaecker (1940), Kimura affirms that for persons with schizophrenia *to be a subject* is not a safe, taken-for-granted possession, rather it is an "endless achievement." This statement comes very close to the ideas of the Italian philosopher and psychopathologist Ernesto De Martino (1997), who argued that in the schizophrenic world being present or being there is a reality to-be-built (*realtà condenda*). The achievement character of "to be" for persons with schizophrenia makes them live in the temporal mode of the *gerundive* ("condenda" in Latin means "due to be built"). Being-there is always in the making, it is an endless task. A schizophrenic person, like the skeptical or transcendental philosopher, is a perennial beginner. Like such traditional philosophers (and contrary to some of their pragmatic or science-inflated contemporary heirs), the schizophrenic lacks the ground for a stable and untroubled being, that is, a proportionate articulation between being rooted in the past and projected into the future. The ground for a secure being is for all of us our rootedness in our own past, our acquaintance with ourselves, and our familiarity with our own environment.

Major schizophrenic symptoms (e.g. thought insertion, hallucinations, or passivity experiences) can be regarded as manifesting a disturbance of the constitutive synthesis of time consciousness. With the fracturing of the time flow, we observe an *itemization* of now-moments in consciousness, so that each now-moment in a person's stream of consciousness will be experienced as detached from the previous one and from the following, hence as extraneous to one's stream of consciousness and sense of selfhood. In schizophrenia, a collapse of the very vector-like nature of the present moment occurs; as a result, rather than merely experiencing time flow as slowing (as is the case with major depression) or accelerating (mania), life itself can turn into a series of stills as time turns wholly strange and unpredictable. Unlike in major depression, in which the crisis of life-drive that projects into the future leaves the person dominated by the past, in schizophrenia, temporality may lose all organization and meaning.

All this seems to suggest that persons affected by these abnormal temporality experiences are unable to act or speak in any recognizably temporally coherent way – but this is not the case. Even in acute episodes of psychosis patients may still be able to differentiate between the past and the present, or form sentences that are grammatically correct. The reason is that abnormal temporality experiences are not identical to so-called disorders of "objective" time. The latter include disorientation in time (e.g. the inability to correctly tell the time without recourse to a clock), age disorientation, or disorders of chronology. These disorders are often associated with disturbances of consciousness, attention, and memory. Fuchs (2013a, 2013b) proposed a model in which the experience of fragmentation is the core feature of temporality in schizophrenia. In particular, he related schizophrenic disorders of intentionality to the basic temporal structure of consciousness as analyzed by Husserl, assuming that the disturbance may be described as a fragmentation of the intentional arc, which is normally based on passive synthesis or implicit couplings. Passive synthesis is the pre-reflexive unification of impression–retention–protention (see Section 1) – which is essential for our everyday life, since these processes relieve us of the task of actively connecting and building up the perceived objects, situations, and habitual patterns of our life. In schizophrenia the protentional function may be weakened in such a way that the constant intertwining of succeeding conscious moments fails. In addition, this fragmentation may lead to typical schizophrenic phenomena such as loss of spontaneity and hyper-reflexivity, and to full-blown psychotic symptoms such as so-called bizarre delusions and verbal-acoustic hallucinations. So, if the continuity of temporal experience disintegrates (of which abnormal temporality experiences are experiential manifestations), overarching meaningful units are no longer available, thereby creating temporal gaps, e.g. in one's stream of consciousness. In severe cases, thoughts that are no longer embedded in one's stream of thoughts are experienced as, for example, thought interferences, blockages, insertion or withdrawal. These symptoms cannot be explained as a mere disturbance of attention or comprehension at the level of semantic combinations. Rather, the disturbance should be sought at a more basic level where the temporal coherence of conscious awareness is constituted. A failure of the constitutive temporal synthesis may create micro-gaps of conscious experience. Thoughts or other mental phenomena that are no longer embedded in the continuity of basic self-experience may appear in consciousness as "erratic blocks" and experienced as being inserted, or, if further externalized, as auditory hallucinations ("voices"). This coheres with the hypothesis that a breakdown of temporality may be bound up with the breakdown of pre-reflexive self-awareness. As the integration between primal impression–retention–protention is served by working memory (the capacity of maintaining a limited amount of information available for use), an in-depth discussion of these and other neuropsychological functions (e.g. selective attention, preparatory set) as related to the disruption of temporality in schizophrenia is also needed (Fuchs, 2013a).

Abnormal time experience in people with schizophrenia can be characterized as follows:

(1) Disarticulation of time experience

   Patients live the temporal plot as disarticulated. This category includes the following subcategories:

   (a) Disruption of time flow: patients may experience a collection of disarticulated snapshots rather than a coherent series of actions and events (typical sentence: "The world is like a series of photographs").

   (b) Déjà vu/Vecu: patients experience places, people, etc. as already lived; this presupposes a disarticulation between past and present (typical sentence: "When I heard the news I felt I had heard it before").

   (c) Premonitions about oneself: patients live the present as the anticipation of their future, as a forewarning of something that concerns them, e.g. they have a feeling that something is going to happen to them or that they or others are going to do something (typical sentence: "I have a premonition of what is going to happen to myself").

   (d) Premonitions about the external world: patients live the present as the anticipation of their future, as a presentiment about the external world (e.g. they experience that something is going to happen in the external world) (typical sentence: "Something is going on, as if some drama is unfolding").

(2) Disturbed experience of time speed

   Patients live time speed as disturbed. They can live time as decelerated (longer, slower, fixed, frozen), accelerated, or both decelerated and accelerated (typical sentences are: "I felt I was moving normally and everyone was moving slowly"; "Time went by very quickly"; "Mouth movement and speech of others are out of synchronization: one faster and the other slower").

(3) Discrepancies about time experiences

   Patients live time "differently" compared to their previous or common-sense experience of time, or they feel themselves lost regarding the common temporal references (typical sentences: "Time is somewhat changed"; "Time isn't supposed to be the way it was. I don't know in what way. I have to think about it").

Lived Space

Changes in the perception of things and space are not infrequent in schizophrenia. Jaspers already mentioned space (and time) as a primary and omnipresent element in the sense world of human beings: "Space seemed to stretch and go on into infinity, completely empty. I felt lost, abandoned to the infinities of space, which in spite of my insignificance somehow threatened me" (Jaspers, 1997: 81).

In schizophrenia, lived space is no longer a space of possibility within whose extension one feels able to "reach" things in the world. Rather, lived space in schizophrenia is a kind of *espace figé* (Callieri, 1999). In this kind of space, things may not appear meaningfully related to one's own body. This phenomenon is related to the abnormality of emotional engagement. People with schizophrenia may find themselves living in a strange and uncanny space, at times dull, at times infinite and limitless. Also, the schizophrenic space is one where objects are flat, or fragmented. Patients try to describe these quasi-ineffable experiences using generic terms as "unreal," "inscrutable," "fake," "meaningless," and define their condition as characterized by "disorientation," "bewilderment," "incertitude," "awe," and so on.

Disorders of lived space in schizophrenia may be classified into four main categories:

(1) Loss of perspectival properties

One key feature of lived space in schizophrenia is its growing homogeneous, two-dimensional nature, losing its perspectival quality. Space appears as a rarefied atmosphere, shaded or fuzzy, or an extension with blinding light. It seems that patients lose their sense of having any subjective center at all, a point of view, or orientation. It may involve an ineffable feeling of being surrounded by unknown territories. Also, the background of lived space can be experienced as coming into the foreground as lived space loses its perspectival quality and paradoxically becomes an unfathomed flatness. This uncanny experience of flatness is taken by the patient as an intimation and a warning: what appears is mere surface, façade, exteriority – a mask hiding a baffling profundity (typical sentences: "There is only the space between things; things are there in a fashion but not so clear"; "I felt spaceless").

(2) Itemization

Another typical feature is the fragmentation of space *Gestalt* reducing the ensemble of a living situation to a mere collection of itemized details. Space is reduced to a disarticulated collection of unrelated items, or decontextualized details (typical sentences: "In the silence and immensity, each object was cut off by a knife, detached in the emptiness, in the boundlessness, spaced off from other things"; "I am overwhelmed by too much detail – too much detail in objects").

(3) Alteration of spatial properties of things

Often anomalies in lived space are described by patients, rather than as anomalies of space itself, as anomalies in the way things appear in space. This category includes various types of anomalous experiences, such as alteration of dimensions and shape of objects, e.g. macropsia, micropsia, and dysmegalopsia, objects fragmented, flat, or unrelated (typical sentences: "For a while it seemed big and open, then too close to me"; "My perception of the world seemed to sharpen the sense of the strangeness of things"; "The air was between things, but the things themselves were not there").

(4) Centrality

Things, persons, situations, and events are experienced as being related to or directed at oneself (self-reference). These feelings may stem from the behavior or the physiognomy of other persons, or from things in the environment. Conrad (1966) uses the term *anastrophé* to capture this self-referential, introversive, or self-observing quality that usually paves the way to the formation of delusions. The patient experiences the world as somehow insinuating and referring to himself. *Anastrophé* is strictly related to apophany (literally: revelation) – an abnormal, sometimes excruciating sense of meaningfulness that can affect "internal" (body, stream of consciousness) as well as "external space." The patient attributes these changes to the external world and searches for clues to render the new unpredictable changes more comprehensible (typical sentences: "The handkerchief on the scaffolding was a message telling me something"; "People were following me around").

Lived Body

Since disorders of the embodied self may be a privileged vantage point to understand the schizophrenic experiences, achieving a detailed clinical characterization of abnormal bodily experiences is essential. Indeed, the weakening of the basic sense of self, the disturbance of implicit bodily functioning, and the disruption of intercorporeal (i.e. body-to-body) resonance are related to fundamental disturbances of emotionality, i.e. self-affection and attunement. Notably, although these concepts might appear distant and obsolete in contemporary operational psychiatry, the notions of cenesthesia and cenesthopathy have been central for the conceptualization of aberrant somatosensory experiences since the early days of psychopathological research in the late nineteenth century. For example, Wernicke emphasized the bodily topicality of "vital feelings," Glatzel described several varieties of disturbances of bodily feelings (*Leibgefuhlsstörungen*), and Jaspers assigned to the awareness of the body an important role for "personalization" (i.e. the I-quality of experience). Later, Huber (1957) described a subtype of schizophrenia primarily characterized by aberrant bodily sensations (i.e. "cenesthopathic schizophrenia"), which maintains a considerable clinical appeal even today. Nonetheless, the concept of cenesthopathic schizophrenia is not recognized as a diagnostic entity in the DSM, and it appears (although relatively undefined) only in the ICD-10.

Patients with schizophrenia frequently present many different kinds of abnormal bodily experiences in the course of their illness, including somatic delusions, coenaesthesias, disturbances of pain perception, out-of-body experiences, dysmorphophobia, body disintegration, and self-injury or self-mutilation. This set of phenomena is heterogeneous and most of them are not specific to schizophrenia.

Most characteristic are ongoing bodily feelings of disintegration/violation and thingness/mechanization. These include experiences of instability of bodily boundaries, externalization of parts of the body that normally are within the bodily boundaries, as well as internalization of objects that normally occupy external space. In addition, fragmentation of bodily construction and changes of body appearance seem also to be typical of schizophrenia. Other typical phenomena are "morbid objectivization" and devitalization. In mainstream clinical scales, abnormal bodily experiences are often listed in the domain of positive symptoms, including somatic delusion, bodily hallucinations, and disorders of ego-boundaries, blurring their specific characteristics and properties. To overcome this problem, ad hoc symptom checklists were designed to assess experiential anomalies in people with schizophrenia that may be considered as subtle and sub- or pre-psychotic disorders (Gross et al., 1987; Parnas et al., 2005). These interviews contain distinct sub-scales for abnormal bodily experiences, but the issue of their sensibility and specificity is still debated.

Summarizing, the characterizing feature of disintegration/violation is a perplexing metamorphosis in one's corporeal borders and *Gestalt*. Patients complain about their body being violated by entities or forces coming from without their own bodily boundaries, e.g. about the intrusion or incorporation of extrapersonal things, forces, and events. Violation typically entails dynamism in the sense of experiencing something moving into oneself, not merely the static presence in oneself of something that should occupy a position external to the self. It also involves experiencing one's body as a thing-like entity, relating to the external world in a mechanical way. Persons with first-episode schizophrenia also experience a dynamization of bodily construction. This is an experience of body disintegration which involves a shifting around of the usual spatial relationships between body parts, or a dynamic distortion of body *Gestalt*, i.e. of one's body as a unitary and integrated structure. Parts of the body are felt as moving away from their usual position. As in the experience of violation, one's body is felt as a spatialized thing-like entity functioning in a quasi-mechanical way. A third aspect of bodily dynamization is the experience of externalization, that is, feeling one's body or parts of it projected beyond one's ego boundaries into the outer space. As is the case with violation and distortion of body construction, externalization is not a static experience but it implies movement. Ego and corporeal boundaries, so to say, are violated from within by parts of the body that are felt as expelled into the outer space. In this type of experience as well, parts of one's body are experienced as thing-like entities in an outer space.

The characterizing feature of thingness/mechanization is an uncanny morbid objectivization and devitalization of the body or its parts. In morbid objectivization, parts of one's body that are usually silently and implicitly present and at work become explicitly experienced. Typically, morbid objectivization goes together with the experience of devitalization, that is, parts of one's body are felt as devoid of life and/or substituted by some kind of mechanism. In general, the body or its parts are experienced as mere things, thing-like or corpse-like entities, rather than as living flesh. Parts of oneself are spatialized – experienced as if they were disintegrated from the living totality of one's body.

There are four categories of abnormal bodily phenomena (Stanghellini, Ballerini, et al. 2015):

(1) Dynamization

This category refers to the way patients experience their bodily boundaries and construction. Dynamization includes three subcategories:

(a) Dynamization of bodily boundaries. Patients report the perplexing experience of strange, uncommon forces or objects violating from outside the boundaries of the body. A typical sentence is: "Areas of body where forces enter."

(b) Dynamization of bodily construction. Patients report perplexing phenomena of unusual, strange movements or forces acting inside one's body; bodily components are also experienced as moving away from their usual position, shifting around the usual spatial relationships. A typical sentence is: "Mouth was where hair should be."

(c) Externalization. Bodily components, vital energies, or biological activities are experienced as projected beyond one's somatic boundaries. A typical sentence is: "Vagina half outside."

(2) Morbid objectivation

This category refers to the way persons experience the vitality and workings of their body. Patients explicitly perceive bodily parts or functions that are typically in the tacit background of experience. There is an increased degree of "thingness" in the body. Parts of oneself are spatialized, as if they were not part of the living body. Also, the body is experienced as devoid of life or substituted by some kind of mechanism. A typical sentence is: "I felt programmed like a robot."

(3) Dysmorphic-like phenomena

This category refers to the way patients experience and represent the external form and appearance of their body. This category includes two subcategories:

(a) Dysmorphic phenomena. This includes puzzling phenomena of an ongoing change/destructuring in parts of one's body, especially its form/appearance, or in the body as a whole; the experience may involve the entire organism, or components. A typical sentence is: "My nose is changing."

(b) Dysmorphophobia. Patients are puzzled about the form/appearance of their body because they experience it as ugly, or having some physical defect (especially asymmetry or change in proportion), although they appear to others within normal limits. A typical sentence is: "Bust bigger and bones smaller."

(4) Pain-like phenomena

This is a residual category that may also include phenomena that are not specific to schizophrenia. The core phenomenon in this category is that the patients report unpleasant/painful bodily feelings that are not substantiated by any medical evaluation; experiences may present themselves in the form of paroxysms or persistent sensations; they are characterized by feelings of strangeness. A typical sentence is: "Pains and feelings of being cut up in various parts of the body."

Self

The disruption in the basic sense of being a self is another fundamental feature in schizophrenia. The level of basic self-awareness in schizophrenia had previously come into view (Berze and Gruhle, 1929) as a diminished state of awareness or mental activity which was called hypophrenia. Minkowski (1927) also developed concepts of the schizophrenic core disturbance as a loss of vital contact to reality. But it was not until the 1960s that Huber and his group reactivated these approaches by their concept of "basic symptoms," later to be extended by Klosterkoetter's investigations of the transitions from basic to full-blown psychotic symptoms (Huber, Gross, and Schüttler, 1979; Huber, 1983, 1995; Klosterkoetter 1988, 1992).

Recently, after several decades of neglect, the concept of "selfhood" assumed again relevance for understanding and diagnosis of schizophrenia spectrum disorders. Drawing on Michel Henry's concept (1973) of the basic sense of existing and the philosopher Michael Polanyi's notion of the "tacit dimension" – together with various ideas from Husserl and Merleau-Ponty – Sass and Parnas (2003) have interpreted schizophrenia as a disorder of the pre-reflexive self, i.e. a pervasive perturbation of the core sense of self or self-affection that is normally implicit in each act of awareness. These changes in the basic structures of consciousness are accompanied by an alteration of the very structure of the field of awareness, which leads to an emergent, particular way of experiencing that is infused by: (a) a change in the focus or salience with which objects and meanings emerge from the background context; (b) an altered conceptual "grip" or "hold" on the world; (c) a mutual amplification of the growing dissolution of the sense of existing as a subject with a more pronounced, disturbing, and alienating self-scrutiny; and (d) an increasing objectification and externalization of normally tacit inner phenomena, with a morbid objectification of one's own psychic life. At the extreme of such progression the person might lose the naturally pre-given sense of coinciding with his own thoughts, sensations, and actions and may feel that he is under the influence of some alien force or entity. We may distinguish two main domains of self-disorders in schizophrenia:

(1) Diminished self-affection

This refers to the breakdown of the crucial sense of self-sameness, of existing as a unified, unique, and embodied subject of experience that is at one with oneself at any given moment. When this basic sense of self is disturbed, the person is inclined to experience a concomitant fading in the tacit, pre-verbal feeling of existing as a living and unified subject of awareness and a kind of exaggerated self-consciousness (hyper-reflexivity, see below). Self-affection provides to subjective experience the sense (pre-reflexive) of being the owners (mineness) and initiators (agency) of our own thoughts, behaviors, and emotions. Experiences of intra-psychic and somato-psychic depersonalization emerge in the split between parts of one's self. Typical sentences: "I feel my self dislocated from its normal position"; "I do not feel my self anymore."

(2) Hyper-reflexivity

Diminished self-affection is associated with a complementary tendency towards focal awareness of aspects of consciousness and the body that would normally be experienced in a tacit or immediate manner. Hyper-reflexivity may occur in an "operative," automatic, or non-volitional fashion. It emphasizes the capacity of the self to split into a subject and an object of experiences and implies, e.g. the perceptualization of inner speech or thought. Typical sentences: "I had to think about what to think"; "I can feel my thoughts as they come out of my mind."

Otherness

Another dimension of the basic structures of subjectivity, essential for the reconstruction of the life-world of the persons with schizophrenia, is the difficulty of entering into contact with other persons.

Social dysfunction (DSM's Criterion B) is a basic diagnostic criterion and a specific and autonomous psychopathological dimension of schizophrenia. It comprises a set of related dysfunctions that contribute to define course and outcome. There are three main limitations of the concept of social dysfunction: (1) it endorses a strictly behavioral-functionalist perspective in which deficits in social behavior are emphasized; (2) these deficits are mainly defined and assessed in terms of quantitative reduction of performance; (3) it encompasses too many heterogeneous domains of life, e.g. everyday functioning, social contacts, education, occupation, and consequences of stigmatization. As a consequence of these limitations, it is difficult (if not impossible) to distinguish social dysfunction in schizophrenia from social dysfunction in other psychopathological syndromes, or social dysfunction that merely emerges in the face of adversity. The main shortcoming of most studies on social dysfunction in schizophrenia reflects these limitations since they do not properly investigate the personal level of experience in real-world functioning. In classical psychopathology, "autism" is the most famous construct depicting both the detachment in schizophrenia from social milieu and their constitution of a private world either filled out by efflorescent imaginative inner life or emptied in a cold rarefaction leaving behind only odd and aloof simulacra (Stanghellini and Ballerini, 2004). Introduced by Eugen Bleuler, autism was conceived as a defense mechanism for managing the conflicts between desires and reality testing. It was described as disengagement from everyday activities, emotional indifference, inappropriate behaviors, and dereistic and overinclusive thinking. In a more phenomenological-experiential vein, Kretschmer (1921/1961) depicted autism in schizophrenia as an emotional paradox: a form of emotional ataxia whose main features are coldness, lack of affective contact with other persons combined with irritability and hypersensitivity to social stimuli, social anxiety and avoidant behavior. Modern accounts of autism mainly draw on Minkowski's (1927) and Blankenburg's (1969) conceptualizations. Minkowski assumed that autism in schizophrenia is a loss of vital contact with reality. Vital contact with reality provides a latent awareness of reality "making us adjust and modify our behavior in a contextually relevant manner but without distorting our overall goals, standards and identity" (Urfer, 2001: 282). Blankenburg characterized autism as a crisis of "common sense": the lack of an implicit understanding of the axioms of everyday life (the background of tacit knowledge shared by a social group, through which its members conceptualize objects, situations, and other persons' behaviors) and of the natural attitude (being attuned to the world as it appears in everyday experience). The fundamental anomaly is understood to be in our preconceptual and pre-cognitive grip on social situations, a kind of pre-reflexive "indwelling" in the social world.

The concept of "schizophrenic autism" (which has apparently vanished from mainstream psychiatry) addresses the core or essential and stable psychopathological nucleus characterizing the quality of dyssociality in persons with schizophrenia. The concept of autism is not limited to aspects of quantitative behavioral deficits, but it also includes phenomena qualitatively defined as anomalous emotional attunement, the tendency to rumination not oriented towards reality, adherence to idiosyncratic ideas, and an unusual hierarchy of values, aims, and ambitions. In particular, the neglect of the value system of persons suffering from schizophrenia contributes to seeing them merely as people who behave inappropriately and who have pathological experiences and beliefs; this may have a stigmatizing effect on them and contribute to judging some of these people's actions as meaningless and incomprehensible. The core feature of schizophrenic autism lies in a specific kind of disorganization of the basic structures of social life – the qualitative disturbance of spontaneous and intuitive participation in social life, i.e. of the emotional conative-cognitive human ability to perceive the existence of others as similar to one's own, make emotional contact with them and intuitively access their mental life. The phenomenon of autism concerns a fundamental aspect of existence: the ability to take part in social life, giving a sense to others' behaviors and to one's existence according to the horizon of meanings of the world surrounding us. The phenomenon of autism implies a fracture in social life, which is therefore compromised in both: (1) the ability to recognize others as individuals endowed with complex and interrelated mental states (emotions, thoughts, feelings of affection which influence one another) having a structure basically similar to our own, and (2) the possibility to understand other people by means of pre-reflective and non-propositional attunement with the expressions of their mental life and by means of a keyboard of shared symbols and experiences. The emotional capability to view others as people like ourselves, to establish interpersonal relations with them intuitively and spontaneously, and the ability to communicate according to common codes: together, the social world as horizon of one's own initiatives and one's own plans for life, undergoes, through autism, a paradoxical distortion.

Starting from considerations stated earlier, it is possible to identify five distinctive categories that characterize the world of schizophrenic autism (Stanghellini and Ballerini, 2004; Stanghellini, Ballerini, et al., 2014).

(1) Hypo-attunement

This is the immediate feeling of reduced attunement, i.e. emotional contact and detachment from other persons, and the pervasive feeling of inexplicable incomprehensibility of people's behaviors and social situations. It includes:

(a) Immediate feeling of distance detachment or lack of resonance. An immediate feeling of distance and detachment, a sense of barrier between oneself and the other. Typical sentence: "I always felt as if I belonged to another race."

(b) Immediate feeling of incomprehensibility of other people and social situations. The lack of intuitive "grip" on social situations. Typical sentence: "I simply cannot grasp what others do."

(c) Ego-syntonic feelings of radical uniqueness and exceptionality. The exaltation of one's feelings of radical uniqueness and exceptionality. It seems to be grounded in anomalous sensations, feelings of disconnectedness from commonly shared reality. Typical sentence: "I've always thought myself to be radically different from all other people, perhaps an alien. It depends on all my strange thoughts which surprised me."

(2) Invasiveness

This is the feeling of being oppressed and invaded by the others, from without. It includes:

(a) Immediate feeling of hostility or oppression. The experience of being invaded, flooded by the external world or by other people, or being somehow in a passive, dangerously exposed position. Typical statement: "I feel driven by the human flood. It is a feeling of danger, as if I were invaded."

(b) Immediate feeling of lack of self-other boundaries. An immediate feeling of being somehow "too open or transparent," of being physically invaded or penetrated by other people's gestures, speech, actions, or glances. Typical statement: "I feel people entering inside me."

(c) Hyper-empathic experiences. The inability to take distance from other people determined by immediate feelings of merging with other persons, direct mindreading of others, fusional, or mimetic experience. Typical sentence: "I feel the mental states of others and I can no longer find myself."

(3) Cenesthopathic/emotional flooding

This is the feeling of being oppressed and submerged from within by paroxysms of one's emotions and bodily sensations evoked by interpersonal contacts. It includes:

(a) Emotional paroxysms. Feeling overloaded by one's distressing emotions in the form of paroxysms when in front of others. Typical sentence: "When people get too close to me I feel tension in my muscles."

(b) Coenesthesic paroxysms. Feelings of being oppressed by uncanny and incomprehensible bodily sensations evoked by interpersonal contacts. Typical statement: "When I look someone straight in the eyes I feel strange vibrations inside."

(4) Algorithmic conception of sociality

This is a conceptual, analytic, hyper-cognitive, hyper-rationalist, hyper-reflective stance towards sociality and the adoption of a "mathematizable" conceptualizations of interpersonal transactions in everyday life. Its main features are:

(a) Observational (ethological) attitude: the attempt to make sense of the mental states of others that lie behind their behavior through empirical observations of other people in everyday life transactions, or from the "scientific" analysis of the workings of "intelligent" mechanisms. Typical statement: "I study people. I am curious. I want to understand how they are inside."

(b) Algorithmic conception of sociality: the observational attitude provides the basis for developing an explicit personal method or algorithm to take part in social transactions. Typical statement: "I have studied a system to intervene at the right moment in conversations."

(5) Antithetic attitude towards sociality

An antithetic attitude towards sociality is the value-structure or existential orientation of persons with schizophrenia. It includes:

(a) Antagonomia: the feeling of being vulnerable to the influx coming from the external world and the claim of one's independence as the most important value. Conventional (common-sense) assumptions, social-shared knowledge, common ways of thinking and behaving and immediate (empathic) relationships and emotional attunement are evaluated as dangerous sources of loss of individuation. Typical statement: "What I detest more is being persuaded by others."

(b) Abstract idealization: replacing the engagement with "real" persons by a marked utopian interest in mankind or abstract humanitarian values. Typical statement: "I love Mankind, but I detest humans."

(c) Idionomia: a kind of exalted existential standpoint that does not allow integration or compromise with the other's point of view or with common sense. Idionomia is comprehensive of metaphysical concerns (they are skeptical about the face value of phenomena) and charismatic concerns (they are convinced that they have a mission to accomplish). Typical statements: "I must test the reality of reality"; "Through suffering, from God I will have the power over the planet."

Values

To persons affected by schizophrenia, the world of human beings may appear undecipherable, its "code" uncrackable. How human beings are able to successfully interact with each other, reciprocally understand each other, how they comprehend the current situation, and make plans together – all seems mysterious. The following sentences are quite significant in this sense:

- "Reality is too complex, and I can't find the key rules."
- "I'd like to graft a file of discourses onto my memory which I could pull up at the right time."
- "I feel inadequate and it's such a pain – I have to come up with algorithms to go and talk with some guy."
- "I lack the backbone of rules of social life. I've spent whole afternoons at parks observing how others interact with each other."

What emerge from these statements are: (1) perplexity, amazement, and a feeling of being extraneous to the social world; (2) the lack of an implicit, spontaneous, and unmediated basis for their own social behaviors; (3) an attempt at filling this lack of intuitive and spontaneous attunement by discovering (or sometimes building) an explicit algorithm, elaborated from observation of the human world and applied in a mediated way; and (4) a mechanistic, and in some way "mathematizable" conceptualization of the phenomenon of intersubjectivity. In other words, this can be translated as a *breakdown of common sense*. Indeed, common sense functions as the fundamental bond that links each individual to the social world; it is the genuine milestone and condition for the possibility of social life (Stanghellini, 2000b, 2001; Stanghellini and Ballerini, 2002). Schizophrenia involves a profound alteration of common sense, i.e. of the symbolic register of socially shared meanings and of pre-reflexive I–You attunement. Both the feeling of perplexity, i.e. the depths of doubt that occur during the initial phases of schizophrenia, and the deviated behavior during the pre-morbid period can be seen as an expression of a crisis of partici-pation in common sense. The loss of the reassuring participation in socially shared interpretive procedures leads to the inability to understand the meaning of the objects that occupy one's own cultural context, the sets of regulations required by social situations. All this takes on a totally different value for people suffering from schizophrenia, compared with healthy people.

Common sense is a framework that disposes a person towards certain values and a context that serves to structure such values. Eccentric values in persons with schizophrenia are one aspect of an overall crisis of common sense; the outcome of this has been designated as antagonomia and idionomia. Let us have a closer look at these two phenomena.

Antagonomia (literally: striving against rules) is often linked with a type of socialization anomaly, namely heteronomic vulnerability. Whereas heteronomic vulnerability reflects the immediate experience of the Other as an overwhelming entity that may jeopardize my own sense of selfhood, antagonomia reflects the axiological dimension of this phenomenon. Antagonomia is the cornerstone of the value system of persons with schizophrenia; it is a cognitive requirement, it is the "philosophy of life" that can be made explicit in propos-itional terms, followed as a guideline of one's actions and, more generally, of the plan for life that each of us strives to carry out. In other words, antagonomia reflects the choice to distance oneself from common-sense rules and take an eccentric stand in the face of commonly shared assumptions and the here-and-now "other."

Idionomia reflects the sentiment of the radical uniqueness and exceptionality of one's own internal law (nomos) with respect to common sense or other human beings. This may go together with an appreciation of one's own radical exceptionality, which is felt as a "gift," often in view of an eschatological mission or a vocation to a superior, novel, metaphysical understanding of the world.

We assume that antagonomia and idionomia in persons with schizophrenia form a structure that is rooted in the person's ontological constitution. The problem, in this vein, is that we need to see what is the connection between values and the essential character of the ontological constitution – i.e. the ontological insecurity (Laing, 2010) and eccentricity (Stanghellini and Ballerini, 2007) of persons with schizophrenia.

Based on patients' personal accounts, the schizophrenic value system emerges as an overall crisis of common sense whose main features are the following (Stanghellini and Ballerini, 2007):

(1) Ego-syntonic feelings of radical uniqueness and exceptionality

Persons with schizophrenia feel "detached from (commonly shared) reality" and "away from home"; they claim to be "radically different from all other people" and "exceptional." Their sentiment of exceptionality is apparently rooted in strange sensations (e.g. "I feel strange energies"; "[I feel] perhaps an alien or an evil creature"), experiences of disconnection from commonly shared reality (e.g. "In my head there is the time zone of California"; "I would be away from home in any part of the world"), and quasi-solipsistic feelings of being the creator of one's own reality (e.g. "I live from the reality I am able to build"; "I don't perceive anymore what I feel, but what I imagine"). These strange phenomena are not felt as merely disturbing or alienating but are ego-syntonically embedded in the person's narrative identity as a gift or a privilege ("This does not happen to every-one!" "It's a privilege"). They are the source of extremely relevant questions, inquiry, and speculations; these feelings of radical exceptionality are frequently integrated in the value system of persons with schizophrenia and may be meaningfully connected to their characteristic metaphysical concerns ("I am a psychoparanoid detached from reality. One of these days someone should explain to me what reality really is"), as is addressed in the next feature.

(2) Metaphysical concerns, including ontological, anthropological, and semantic concerns

Persons with schizophrenia are not satisfied with what appears in immediate experience and are concerned with metaphysical questions. These questions are chiefly ontological. Ontology (from ont – being and logos) is the theory of being, the discourse about things that constitute reality and especially about their "being," i.e. their existence (vs. non-existence) and their true meaning (vs. ordinary meaning). Ontology, as a branch of philosophy, deals with a series of conceptual dichotomies like appearance/ actuality, necessity/contingency, permanence/transience, singularity/universality, substance/accident, identity/diversity, etc. It is essentially concerned with questions like what really exists, in contrast with what only seems to exist. What exists independently and unconditionally, in contrast to what exists dependently and conditionally? What permanently exists, in contrast to what only temporarily exists? Persons with schizophrenia are especially explicitly concerned with the first question (e.g. "I must test the reality of reality"). The following sentence epitomizes the ontological attitude: "My attitude towards life can be summed up as follows: It is as if we were all at theater. But, whereas, all the others are focused on what happens on the stage I cannot help thinking of what's going on backstage, what makes the scene possible." They observe everyday, pragmatic reality from without (e.g. "I am like an emperor in a pyramid. I am not involved in the world, merely observing it from outside to understand its secret workings"; "I am a detached onlooker"), engaged in understanding its workings either being skeptical about the face value of phenomena (e.g. "It is not enough for me to take things as the others do") or feeling unable to unreflectively grasp their meaning (e.g. "The others know the rules; I have to study them"). Many persons with schizophrenia report that they feel like anthropologists, as if they were coming from another planet (e.g. "I am like an anthropologist"; "I am an anthroponaut lost at sea"). Human actions and interactions are their focus of concern and research (e.g. "I like to get walking around. I am fascinated by observing other people in everyday activity and seeing how it functions"). Also, persons with schizophrenia may be unsatisfied with ordinary semantics for articulating their own way of experiencing the world (e.g. "I don't understand why this has to be called a table, and if the sun's out we have to say it's a nice day") and look for alternative means of expression (e.g. "I will use my left hand for writing in order to activate a new part of my brain").

(3) Charismatic concerns

The sentiment of radical uniqueness and exceptionality of persons with schizophrenia may entail their feeling gifted (charisma originally means gift, although in ordinary language it has the connotation of "emotionally compelling" or "attractive") with superior spiritual powers (e.g. "I have this spiritual level"; "I have the invention in my head"). They feel chosen for an important eschatological (eschatos means "ultimate") task (e.g. "I was chosen for this. Something extremely important") and committed to use their privilege to save mankind from evil (e.g. "I was given this task from God: the fight between good and evil"; "I have a mission, I should look for the Devil"), to build a better and more authentic world (e.g. "To build a more livable and fraternal world"; "I walk downtown in Florence watching the most important monuments meanwhile I dictate how to improve them"), or a deeper understanding of reality (e.g. "I was given some powers from God to penetrate the deep sense of reality"), or of other people (e.g. "I made my senses more sensible to feel the Holy Spirit of people"). Thus, the sufferings, detachment from reality, desertification of the world, and uncanny sensations of persons with schizophrenia get the character of a charisma (e.g. "Through suffering from God I will have the power over the planet. This will happen as soon as all people disappear from the world. It will be a desert planet, I will be able to pass from one temporal dimension to another, I will meet only replicas of myself"). There is an in-order-to quality of a commitment or a value, i.e. of a set of motivational feelings, rooted in the person's ontological constitution, that serves as the criterion for preferring and acting in a given way.

(4) Refusal of interpersonal bonds

Next to these feelings of detachment from commonly shared reality and from other people, we find the deliberate choice to distance oneself from the here-and-now "other." Being disconnected and the refusal of intimate interpersonal connections often coexist (e.g. "I cannot reach them but I also don't want to reach them"; "I am not able to take part in the world as the others and I don't like it"). Interpersonal bonds are rejected (e.g. "Interpersonal bonds have no reason to exist") and one's own tendency to identify with others is especially feared (e.g. "I reject my tendency towards identifying myself with what the others say"; "What I detest more than anything else is being persuaded by others"). The contact with other human beings may be felt as a dangerous source of loss of identity (e.g. "I'm getting to be more humane. Will it ruin my brain? All this humanity is upsetting my own special framework. It's polluting me") or original thought (e.g. "I would like to be clearheaded to have intuitions. And for this I would like not to be too domesticated"). Detachment and feeling different from others are acknowledged as positive values (e.g. "I feel all right on my own"; "I've always liked being different very much").

(5) Refusal of common-sense knowledge and semantics

The last feature of the value system of persons with schizophrenia is their choice to distance themselves from common-sense rules and take an eccentric stand in the face of conventional meanings, values, beliefs, and ordinary ways to convey them – all this epitomized in the sentence "My aversion to common sense is stronger than my instinct to survive." Essential features of the value system of persons with schizophrenia are a disdainful refusal of the ordinary way of being and the taken-for-granted understanding of reality (e.g. "Man is merely a heap of memories in a standard hardware"; "The brain is

Table 14.1 The values of persons with schizophrenia

Values

1. Ego-syntonic feelings of radical uniqueness and exceptionality

2. Metaphysical concerns, including ontological, anthropological, and semantic concern

3. Charismatic concerns

4. Refusal of interpersonal bonds

5. Refusal of common-sense knowledge and semantics

a believalogical imbecile"), a skeptical attitude towards conventional knowledge (e.g. "Mathematics, geometry, art, and justice, are the improper certainties of human beings"; "Objectivity is the involution of subjectivity"), a praise of disconnectedness and an attempt at bracketing common sense to get a deeper understanding of reality (e.g. "Revelation is a subjective vision of the human condition disconnected from the 'common' idea to be or to belong to the human condition"; "Madness is necessary to human intelligence to get to the higher levels"). Sometimes, this rejection of common sense and "objective" knowledge is part of a more general clash between oneself as a "different" and unique person and the other human beings that are felt as a dangerous source of loss of individuality (e.g. "Civilization is objectivity made common by the incompatibility of subjectivities"; "By being by myself I am able to understand that nothing has a sense"). Common sense, the tacit codex that implicitly allows human beings to understand each other, is at the same time lacking and rejected (e.g. "I admitted the physiological abjuration of common sense, in the moment in which I could admit the desperate effort to understand the tacit codex that is implicit in human actions"). A skeptical attitude also involves conventional semantics. Its main characteristics are criticizing the usual object–meaning pairing allowed for by common sense and the attempt to devise better tools to express one's own often idiosyncratic experiences (e.g. "It's time to change this objective handwriting into a subjective one" [written in a diary where the handwriting goes on with an idiosyncratic alphabet]).

Table 14.1 summarizes the values of persons with schizophrenia.

Conclusion

Persons with schizophrenia convey an appreciation and often an exaltation of their own feelings of radical uniqueness and exceptionality. Sometimes, all this is claimed as the result of a free choice, the effect of a "diverse will." Indeed, it can be assumed that the value system of schizophrenic persons is centered on a deliberate epistemological and ethical attitude consisting in the disdainful refusal of taken-for-grantedness of conventional meanings, values, and beliefs. Persons with schizophrenia are purposely oriented towards being against the ordinary mode of existence.

Choice and necessity cannot be easily disentangled. From another angle, the schizophrenic person's lack of common sense can be seen as a destiny, an ontological necessity, and not a lifestyle choice. Their claim to be "radically different from all other people" (category 1) is seemingly rooted in a profound metamorphosis of self-awareness. Parts of the self are objectified, spatialized, i.e. felt as existing in an outer space. For instance, thoughts may be experienced as existing somewhere outside the limits of what defines the self, and persons may feel thrown away from their natural seat and can only contemplate themselves from the outside or from a third-person perspective. In this state, there is a loss of pre-reflexive, immediate self-awareness, including the feeling of agency (the sense that it is I that is the source of this thought or movement) and of ownership or myness (the sense that it is I who am experiencing this thought, emotion, or movement as my own). The sentiment of exceptionality is grounded in anomalous sensations, feelings of disconnectedness from commonly shared reality, and solipsistic experiences.

Values are embedded in a context – a world – that is quite different from the common-sense world. The feeling of ontological eccentricity (transformation of self–world relationship) is the core value in persons with schizophrenia. This core value or ur-value is not an articulate concept; rather it is an evaluative attitude that arises from a special kind of self–world transformation. It is basically a given, not a choice, and the source of the characteristic charismatic and metaphysical concerns in persons with schizophrenia. Binswanger assumed that schizophrenic eccentricity is based on a choice. People with schizophrenia are not eccentric because they try to be different. Their weird behavior is not simply the consequence of an antagonistic lifestyle choice. People with schizophrenia do not strive for being against as such; rather, they strive to be faithful to their own eccentricity, to their own being so. The eccentricity of persons with schizophrenia is a matter of ontology, it is a given, not a lifestyle choice. They are eccentric; therefore, they feel and look different.

Idionomia is originally given in this sentiment and tied up with emotions like "exaltation" and "fascination." Persons with schizophrenia may feel their ontological eccentricity as the supernatural sign of their vocation to an eschatological mission or to a deeper understanding of the world. There are two different ways to react to this feeling of ontological eccentricity: a metaphysical trend (the concern to discover the essence of reality of which other people are ignorant) and a charismatic trend (the concern to use one's own gift to save mankind). Both display that one's own radical exceptionality is positively appreciated and taken as the grounds of an eschatological mission to accomplish. Persons with schizophrenia are captivated by the perplexing metaphysical complexity of existence; their value system reflects this "exalted fascination" for "what is going on in the backstage" and their being disconnected to what appears in immediate experience. Spellbound to ultimate questions and never-ending ontological and anthropological inquiries, persons with schizophrenia lose the "vital" contact with here-and-now reality. Morbid rationalism precisely captures the deliberate epistemological option at work in idionomia, which is an intellectualistic attitude that disparages all skill to shape knowledge in a contextually relevant manner. Also, the concept of "hyper-reflexivity" – i.e. a kind of exaggerated self-consciousness, a tendency to direct focal, objectifying attention towards processes and phenomena that would normally be "inhabited" and thus would not pop up in explicit awareness – nicely portrays the non-intentional, passive side of idionomia.

The most characteristic psychotic symptoms of schizophrenia, i.e. delusions, typically involve idionomia in that they focus on the metaphysical status of reality (and not merely on ontic or empirical-pragmatic issues, like being attacked or conspired against as in persecutory delusions that are not specific to schizophrenia). Typical schizophrenic delusions have as their theme the "being" of the world and its components (including one's own self or parts of it), i.e. their existence (vs. non-existence) and their true meaning (vs. ordinary meaning), and the relationship of knower and known. These typically schizophrenic delusions are deemed "bizarre" because – quoting *DSM-5* (2013) – they involve the phenomena that the person's culture would regard as totally implausible and that do not derive from ordinary life experiences.

Idionomia may shed a new light on the bizarreness of bizarre delusions by showing how they arise from a different sort of "being," a radical breakdown of common-sense experiences and understanding of the world (the feeling of ontological uniqueness and exceptionality) and from a coherent set of emotions and values (metaphysical and charismatic concerns) that give rise to the search for a new meaning and a new order of the world itself. In the light of idionomia, bizarreness (including the bizarreness of schizotypal personality disorder, e.g. "odd" beliefs and unusual perceptual experiences) is not simply an incomprehensible deviation from standard behavioral patterns or standard ways of cognition, but the expression of the exalted fascination arising from a radically different kind of being in the world.

Antagonomia reflects the choice to distance oneself from common-sense rules and take an eccentric stand in the face of commonly shared assumptions and the here-and-now "other." In life without psychosis, the understanding of the other is based on a pre-cognitive, intuitive experience, a direct perception of the other's emotional life (so-called primordial intersubjectivity), and on the implicit sharing of a common horizon of meanings (so-called common sense), rather than calculated inferences of others' mental states. Primordial intersubjectivity is the very condition that makes communication possible. Its cornerstone is social attunement, i.e. the affective-cognitive human ability to perceive the existence of others as similar to one's own, make emotional contact with them, and intuitively access their mental life. The sharing of meanings and of social scripts, the understanding of rules, and the adoption of adequate behavioral procedures all depend on the pre-existence of a valid social attunement. Social attunement affords the constitution of common sense. Common sense is the interpretive order valid for every individual belonging to a specific cultural context that makes possible the existence of a socially shared world and pragmatic engagement in it. Every person receives and participates in this interpretive order spontaneously. This implicit sharing is disordered in people with schizophrenia, but it is also rejected. As foreseen by Kretschmer, schizophrenic "disinclination for human society" is seldom mere unfeeling dullness, but it typically involves an "active turning away, of a defensive or more offensive character." Conventional (common-sense) knowledge, immediate (empathic) relationships, and emotional attunement are evaluated as dangerous sources of loss of individuation. As shown by Minkowski, persons with schizophrenia display an antithetical attitude: they feel vulnerable to the influx coming from the external world and claim their independence as the most important value.

The antagonomia concept builds on and extends Minkowski's and Kretschmer's ideas: persons with schizophrenia exhibit a general distrust towards emotional attunement with other people and are skeptical towards conventional knowledge and socially shared values and express an explicit repugnance to common ways of thinking, called "objectivity" or "common sense," and make an attempt at bracketing it. This explicit repugnance towards the pre-reflexive, spontaneous foundations of sociality is apparently in contrast to the authentic interest in others' way of life that appears in the attempt at reflexively building the "algorithms" of social life. Persons with schizophrenia are not uninterested in "real" people; on the contrary, they often do their best to meaningfully connect with them. The social world in schizophrenia thus loses its characteristic as a network of relationships among embodied selves moved by emotions and turns into a cool, incomprehensible game,

Table 14.2 The life-world of persons with schizophrenia

Existential	Experiences
Time	Disarticulation of time experience Disturbed experience of time speed Discrepancies about time experiences
Space	Loss of perspectival properties Itemization Alteration of spatial properties of things Centrality
Body	Dynamization Morbid objectivation Dysmorphic-like phenomena Pain-like phenomena
Other	Hypo-attunement Invasiveness Cenesthopathic/emotional flooding Algorithmic conception of sociality Antithetic attitude towards sociality
Self	Diminished self-affection Hyper-reflexivity
Emotions	Over-sensitive and cold at the same time, although in quite different relational mixtures Trema (a paradoxical mixture of anguish, hope, despair, and suspicion) Crisis of conative-emotional attunement

from which the person feels excluded, and whose meaning is sought through the discovery of abstract algorithms and the elaboration of impersonal rules. The attunement crisis and antagonomia together leave the person with only the third-person perspective from which to characterize and understand the interpersonal world.

Table 14.2 summarizes the life-world of persons with schizophrenia.

The Life-World of Persons with Melancholia

Major depressive disorder is characterized by the heterogeneous symptomatology which affects different domains including affective, cognitive, sensorimotor, and social. Depressed people may feel sad, anxious, empty, hopeless, worried, helpless, worthless, guilty, irritable, or restless. The person may lose interest in activities that were pleasurable; experience loss of appetite or overeating; have problems concentrating, remembering details, or making decisions; and may contemplate, attempt, or even desire suicide. Generally, people affected by major depressive disorder describe their own condition as "living in a black hole" or having a feeling of impending doom. However, some depressed people do not feel sad at all, they may feel lifeless and apathetic, or, in other cases, angry, aggressive, and agitated. In this psychopathological condition, the world appears withered and devoid of freshness and openness.

Depression singular is grammatically misleading. It suggests a well-defined nosographical entity comparable with, say, pneumonia or appendicitis. But depression is heterogeneous at many levels. The boundary between normal sadness and depression is contested. Diagnostic classifications recognize phenomenologically distinct subtypes. There are competing professional models of depressive disorder (medical, psychological, social, and so forth). Above all, and crucially for practice, individual experiences of depression vary widely.

In this chapter, we will focus on one type of depression, namely melancholia. Depression was initially called "melancholia," but "depression" and "melancholia" are not exact expressions for the same phenomenon, although there are similarities. Briefly, the standard use of "depression" refers to a state of more or less intense suffering that generically includes lowered mood, a term whose meaning usually corresponds to "sadness" but that may vary from bad mood (dysphoria) to apathy. The fact that "depressed mood" is conceptually unclear is perhaps the major source of confusion in the classification and understanding of the variety of forms of "depressions."

The term "melancholia," as it is used in phenomenological psychopathology, denotes a special kind of depression characterized by an exacerbated and painful experience of loss of emotional grasp and resonance (Binswanger, 1960; Tellenbach, 1961/1980; Berrios, 1988). It is a special kind of depersonalization characterized by the feeling of the loss of feelings or *not-able-to-be-sad* (*Nichttraurig-sein-Koennen*) – someone who can still be sad is not truly melancholic (Schulte, 1961); it is a degradation of the power for having moods at all (Fernandez, 2016). A paradoxical feature of this experience is that this profound indifference is experienced as a source of suffering. The patient's overall attitude towards this phenomenon is characterized by self-accusing, self-reprimanding, and a sense of guilt. Rarely does the melancholic person limit herself to merely acknowledging her loss of the capacity of feeling; rather her whole experience is permeated by ethical worries. Impaired emotional resonance aggregates with delusions of guilt (Stanghellini and Raballo, 2007). These patients tend to deny retrospectively the authenticity of their own sentiments for others (Kraus, 1994).

As it is clear, "melancholia" denotes a severe depressive episode (Tatossian, 1979, 1983), often associated with psychotic ideas expressing concerns about the consequences of losing moral, financial, or physical integrity (Schneider, 1950; Stanghellini, 2008; Sass and Pienkos, 2013a, 2013b). Furthermore, melancholia is one of the phases of some kinds of manic-depressive ("bipolar") disorder (Binswanger, 1960; Stanghellini and Raballo, 2007).

The aim of this chapter is to describe the life-world of persons affected by this form of depression, linking it with the life-world they used to live in during the pre-morbid or inter-morbid periods of their life.

The Life-World of the Melancholic Type of Personality

The concept of *typus melancholicus* (TM) was shaped by the German psychiatrist Hubertus Tellenbach (1961/1980) to characterize the pre-morbid and inter-morbid personality structure liable to endogenous depression. Tellenbach identified a fundamental set of distinctive features that inform the pre-morbid life-world and lifestyle of persons vulnerable to develop an acute melancholic episode. The work of Tellenbach is essential to clarify the relationship between a pre-morbid personality structure and a typical existential limit situation clinically relevant for the development of an acute melancholic decomposition. By "personality structure" we mean a kind of life-world and a relatively homogeneous set of emotions, values, and social behavior.

Tellenbach's theory is framed by an overarching, global view of man in continuous and essential relationship with the world. This comprehensive view of human existence refers to the concept of *endon* as a way of connection between the psychic and somatic, and between the person and the world. The endogenous indicates the basic biological imprint prior to the formation of the personality, a concept that does not substantially departs from the notion of "emotion" developed in the first part of this book: emotions are embodied functional states that situate a person in the world and protentional states that project the person into the future providing a felt readiness for action (Chapter 8). Indeed, the endogenous is not considered only in relationship with the somatic or psychic sphere, but also includes a notion of the person in his or her relationship with the world. Central in this theory is the role of temporality since all this is directly related to the rhythmic processes of life, that is, to the normal tendency of individuals to adjust and synchronize their biorhythms (sleep, awakeness, etc.) with the world.

Time

This emphasis on temporality is the central feature of all phenomenological theory of the pathogenesis of depression. In normal situations, the rhythmic is understood as a fundamental form of the flow of life, which is expressed in some of the characteristics of human behavior. Rhythm is not a passive reaction to environmental influence; on the contrary, it is the indicator of a natural tendency for synchronization of the person with the world. Both the slowness and speed of a rhythm contribute to the harmony of movement and are a result of a capacity of control and an inner measure.

In pathological conditions, measure and rhythm seem to be absent. Rapidness – understood as swift rhythm – may be replaced by agitation (as is the case with mania), and slowness by delay (as is the case with melancholia). Agreement between subjective and objective rhythm defines a state of harmony. Melancholia may be considered an endogenous condition as it breaks such a harmonic state. Melancholia is linked to *desynchronization* (Fuchs, 2001) between the time of the person and that of the world, in which the world time passes too quickly for the person to catch up with it.

Desynchronization is retardation or acceleration of subjective time in relation to the social sphere. In the life-world of TM persons desynchronization is always incipient. The horror of desynchronization is to the TM the awfulness of falling behind regarding what he deems are the expectations of others. The TM strives not to lag behind his duties and obligation deriving from the social commitments he has taken up. His entire life can be interpreted as an effort to pay his debts before he contracts them. In order to avoid the danger of desynchronization, the TM constantly needs to anticipate what he believes others' requests will be, and timely comply with the duties related to his social roles. For these reasons, he tends to be over-active and over-engaged.

Space

To be over-active and over-engaged is a way to preserve harmony in the social space. In the life-world of TMs, each thing should occupy a dictated place within a pre-established order. Space, in this sense, is not geographical extension, rather a position in social relationships and hierarchies. Things are not mere objects (as is the case with the lived space of the obsessive person), rather other persons. As we will see in more detail analyzing the value-structure of TMs, this typical arrangement of space in social interactions is called "orderliness." The kind of "order" looked for by the TM is not the spatial arrangement of things, but rather assigning a social role to each person (including oneself) in his social environment. Assigning oneself a place is a way to take refuge within the limits of one's order, a defined and limited position within which the TM feels able to exercise her own "autonomy." The need to cling to one's own controllable and predictable order assures the state of well-being and defends from potential threats coming from the world, from the undefined and uncontrollable.

Self-Identity

TMs are affected by a kind of depersonalization involving the process through which we form our identity, that is, the narrative self. The narrative self is the representation one constructs of oneself.

Each person defines his own identity not only according to what he has been, but also based on what he is not-yet, what he could be, and what he would like to be. One's own narrative identity arises from the interplay between I-am's and I-can's. I-can's are what one is not, one's own possibilities. The TM person exiles this duality of existence and inexorably falls into the marsh of merely being-the-same. TM persons insist on a finite and unchosen perspective of stable characteristics that they consider their own, and with which they over-identify. They experience other possibilities merely as a source of alienation or nullification.

Their vulnerability consists in the grinding to a halt of the dialectic between the Self and the Other-than-Self. The Other-than-Self is considered a dangerous source of nullification. In fact, the Other-than-Self is not experienced as a possibility towards which one should reach out, or on the basis of which one could define oneself; it is, instead, experienced as a nothing from which one should run for shelter. This intolerance to other possibilities and the avoidance of the dialectic between I-am's and I-can's immanent in the constitution of one's narrative self leads to an identification with partial, external, and reified identities, namely roll identity, i.e. external/socially appreciated representations of identity. TMs internalize roll identities and through this internalization they acquire a stable, although inflexible, self-identity. Their identity is based on a reified, sclerotic self-representation. It implies an over-simplified categorization of oneself and others, who appear in the light of their social roles, rather than in terms of their ego-identity.

Role identity is that which each person has to assume on the basis of their own social function; self-identity is the self-determination of the personality, that is, beyond simple and straightforward identification with one's role. Distancing from the role is necessary to preserve one's authenticity as a person over and above that of the mere agent of an impersonal role. A person may maintain a sense of autobiographic continuity recognizing herself in spite of the transformation of roll identities and not being vexed by self-alienation and estrangement. Such a vital dialectic between role identity and self-identity is reduced and suppressed in the TM, which tends to collapse and crystallize self-identity in the simulacrum of the role. Indeed, the TM is unable to go beyond the socially established rules, reinterpreting his relation with himself, the Other, and the world in a flexible and autonomous fashion (Ambrosini, Stanghellini, and Langer, 2010).

Other

Just as the TM is unable to perceive himself otherwise than through a social role, so too the Other is always perceived partially, and never as a whole person. The bond with the Other is a bond with the Other's social role (a father, the boss, a doctor, etc.), not a relation with the Other as an individual person. This incapacity to recognize the individuality of the Other is called *idioagnosia*. This bond with the Other *qua* social role serves to reinforce the TM's partial perception of himself as well as to reconfirm himself in a predefined and pre-established role in a tautology of roles that reconfirms itself. The "others" in question for the TM are not the here-and-now, flesh-and-blood others, rather, a sort of generalized Other – the abstract and absolute source and incarnation of impersonal social norms and values. Idioagnosia is blindness to the individuality of oneself and of the Other because persons are perceived solely as generic types.

Idioagnosia leads to *pseudo-intersubjectivity*: TMs' social behaviors are guided neither by personal choice, nor by the finely tuned perception of what the here-and-now Other would choose. Rather, they are guided by standard and anonymous rules and values, like obedience, self-discipline, politeness, etc.

Yet, the TM affirms that he is there *for the Other*. To him, the Other is someone not to be disappointed, to look after, to care for. Social harmony must be preserved at all costs. TM persons can hardly enjoy the pure and simple fact of being with the Other. Their inter-subjectivity does not foresee the implicit pleasure of being together with another. Occupy-ing a place in the physical or relational space is a right to be conquered and earned with effort and determination within a rigid regime of meritocracy. One's moral respectability and accountability are essential prerequisites for engaging in social relationships. In fact, spontaneous free exchanges without any obligation of return are not contemplated; the sense of "justice" is reduced to a circle of *do ut des* (I give and you give back) in which the

TM feels in a position of disadvantage, one step behind. One's autonomy in the practical sense of self-sufficiency, including physical and financial integrity, is needed to avoid any kind of dependence from others.

Emotions

There are three main aspects to the emotional life of TMs: hyperthymia, statothymia, and intolerance of emotional ambiguity.

Hyperthymia

The behavior of TMs is characterized by hyperactivity, over-involvement, and sociability. These traits are part of the temperament of TMs, that is, of the constitutional substratum of their personality, their basic psychic *tempo*. Temperament is the assemblage of habits and skills among which the best validated are emotionality, activity, and sociability (Rutter, 1987; Cloninger, 1994; Jouvent and Widlocher, 1994).

A provocative and apparently counter-intuitive indication is that a predisposing factor for bipolarity, i.e. hyperthymic temperament, is a discriminant trait feature of the TM. Whereas depressive temperament is distributed among all patients who develop major depression, TMs show significantly higher hyperthymic traits as compared to all other categories of patients affected by major depression, the latter mainly showing cyclothymic and irritable traits (Stanghellini, Bertelli, and Raballo, 2006). Especially persons with borderline personality (see Chapter 13) are characterized by the coexistence of an affective cyclothymic temperamental dysregulation with concomitant anxious–dependent traits and by a set of conditions characterized by mood reactivity, interpersonal sensitivity, and enhanced liability to mood, anxiety, and impulse control disorders.

The association of TM and hyperthymic traits is coherent with both idiographical clinical observation by Kretschmer (1921/1961), Lange (1926), Arieti (1959), and Tellenbach (1961), who described hyperactive, eager, and alacritous behaviors in people vulnerable to major depression, and with empirical research into the temperament of major depressives, demonstrating that a significant minority of major depressive "pseudo-unipolar" break-downs arise from a hyperthymic baseline characterized by patterns including highly adaptive extroverted traits, high functioning, tirelessness, enormous capacity for work, and work-addiction, as well as affability, assertiveness, and denial of distress and of personal limitations (Akiskal, 1994, 1996; Perugi et al., 1998; Cassano et al., 1999).

Statothymia

Statothymia, also named *immobilithymia*, is the tendency to cling to a certain mood and therefore to certain ways of being and doing. Persons characterized by statothymia display the same behavioral traits of TMs: they are diligent, honest, scrupulous, and efficient. This characteristic, according to Shimoda (1950), is typical of those structures with the tendency to the development of acute manic-depressive episodes. Statothymia is supposedly a way to cope with the risk of acute episodes representing a functional strategy to prevent manic or depressive decompensation. In contrast to the cyclothymic–anxious–sensitive type, TMs do not show mood lability or impulse dyscontrol as their core feature. The hyperthymic trait usually does not lead TMs to impulsive behavior. Rather, hyperthymia seems to be compensated by the TMs' value-structure (see below) and supports their industriousness, thoroughness, and meticulousness. Indeed, TMs need a lot of energy and vitality to sustain their

Table 15.1 The life-world of *typus melancholicus*

Existential	Experiences
Time	Desynchronization is always incipient Horror of lagging behind
Space	Fixation on order not regarding the spatial arrangement of things, rather assigning a social role to each person in his social environment
Other	Idioagnosia (incapacity to recognize the individuality of the Other) Pseudo-intersubjectivity Being-there for the other
Self	External and reified identities (roll identity), i.e. external/socially appreciated representations of identity
Emotions	Hyperthymia Statothymia Intolerance of emotional ambiguity

conscientious lifestyle. Statothymia seems to contribute to this precarious equilibrium by reinforcing the tendency to hypernomia (see below), perseveration, and to a certain degree of viscosity in their need to maintain the order in their social relations.

Intolerance of Ambiguity

TMs are unable to emotionally tolerate complexity. They cannot cope with the presence of opposite characteristics or dissonant aspects within one situation, even more within the same person (see below). They live, so to say, in a black-and-white world, in which all nuances and gradations of gray are excluded. This incapacity seems to be primarily of an emotional kind: what is intolerable to them is complexity which would jeopardize their world-view, and their own fragile ego-identity, incardinated in an inflexible social order sharply distinguishing what is good from what is bad – obviously overlooking the intricacies of moral aspects within the same person or situation.

Table 15.1 summarizes the life-world of persons with *typus melancholicus*.

Values

TM is a personality structure giving rise to a stable mode of relating to the world and oneself in a way that entails a potential for the development of melancholic episodes. TM is defined by a set of concomitant, stable characteristics that organize their vulnerability and transpire across pre-morbid, inter-morbid, and morbid phases. Crucially, such characteristic imprint is situated at the ethical-ontological level of value-formation. Values pre-structure a world-view that establishes what is relevant and meaningful. In the case of TM, such a world-view already entails a germ of potential decompensation. TMs are basically *centric* persons (Stanghellini, 2000c): hyper-connected to common sense and over-identified with social norms (Kretschmer, 1921/1961; Minkowski, 1927; Tellenbach, 1961/1980; Kraus, 1977). Their style of behavior is impressive for its over-normality, extreme social adjustment, and conformism. The cornerstones of the life-world of TMs are conscientiousness, orderliness, heteronomia, and intolerance of ambiguity.

Conscientiousness

Conscientiousness is the commitment to prevent guilt attributions and guilt feelings in the effort to feel accepted by others (Stanghellini and Bertelli, 2006). Typical statements are "The most important thing for me is a clear conscience," "In order to avoid criticism, I always do my work and if necessary that of the others too," "When I have done something wrong, it always comes back to my mind," "I cannot stand not being at peace with myself."

This is an elevated demand above the mean of one's own possibilities, fueled by the need to prevent feelings and attributions of guilt. TMs aim at fulfilling many obligations, always in a consistent, reliable, and effective way. Clinging to one's own controllable and predictable order assures a state of well-being and defends it from potential threats from the surrounding world, from the undefined and uncontrollable.

Conscientiousness is inspired by a fundamental need to avert any potential feeling of guilt or accusatory attributions. Hence, the TM is constantly seeking acceptance from the Other and his behavior is not based on his own personal criteria, but rather on perceived social expectations. It is important to recognize that the Other in question is not the *here-and-now* Other as an individual person, but the *generalized* Other: the abstract and absolute source of impersonal social norms and values. Conscientiousness is a secularized form of moral conscience. The generalized Other embodies the impersonal values of common sense – what *anyone* thinks and what *anyone* ought to do. It is according to the values that the TM attributes to this impersonal Other that he feels judged and evaluated.

TMs attempt to keep their conscience scrupulously clean. It is fundamental to not be blamed by the Other. Hence, each interpersonal gesture expresses the need to protect oneself from all possibility of loss of the Other's approval.

The idea that the TM has about his or her order does not foresee exceptions, as they are not open to flexible adaptation in accordance with the circumstances. Given that sooner or later, the unforeseen will occur in the scenario of existence, the TM's radical refractoriness to being subject to the unforeseen generates an exposure to vulnerability. In fact, despite the effort in preserving a controlled and ordered existential eco-system, the desired harmony is never a permanent and guaranteed achievement, especially given that the constriction of such rigid limits prevents the TM from developing the necessary transcendence to reach a higher balance. It is as if the TM has acquired once and for all an impersonal order at the cost of sacrificing the margin of subjective freedom that is required to manage their relationship with the world.

Orderliness

Orderliness is defined as the fixation on harmony in interpersonal relationships and the need to avoid conflicts. Typical statements are "I am there for others," "My happiness depends on the happiness of those around me," "I am not able to disagree with others," "I always do my best to be considered a reliable person." Orderliness prevents the possible conflicts that may entail feelings of guilt. TMs try to anticipate any possibility of being in debt. For this purpose, he imposes upon himself an elevated burden of demands and attempts to fulfill obligations in a consistent and steady way.

Orderliness should not be confused with the commitment to maintain the spatial order of things characteristic of obsessive persons. TMs are not primarily interested in the arrangements of objects in space; rather they strive to preserve a pre-established hierarchical order in the social space. Accordingly, to each person is attributed a given social role. TMs continually follow in the footsteps of the faded image of their own existence via an over-identification with their own roll identity. They are extremely dependent on that identity which they find for example in their professional, partner, and other social roles. They over-identify with their social role – which could be that of a devoted son, an affectionate parent, or an honest worker – as well as with the conventional moral values that the role brings with it. According to Kraus (1977, 1982), such an extreme dependence on roll identity is a consequence of a lack of ego-identity and in consequence a lack of ego achievements. This has as a consequence, on the one hand, a rigid behavior in their professional role and, on the other hand, a suppression of all emotions and cognitions which would endanger the identity found in their roles in personal relationships (Kraus, 1977, 1982).

The TM represents a human type ensnared by common sense. He is convinced he seeks for justice and truth, yet his main concerns are order and consensus. The over-identification with tradition is the main characteristic of TM. He submits to the pressure of public opinion, to the icons of identity taken from common-sense stereotypes, and to the gravitational force of social norms as external guidelines for actions.

Heteronomia

Heteronomia (from *hetero* = other and *nomos* = norm, rule) is an exaggerated receptiveness to external norms. Heteronomia is an exaggerated receptivity to standard practice: each action is guided by an impersonal motivation, referring to socially established criteria. It is a kind of ethical hypo-plasticity: TMs adopt pre-established norms that are mainly passively imprinted. Once this normative frame of reference is adopted, TMs are unable to change or transcend it. Heteronomia is significantly linked to *hypernomia*, an excessively rigid adaptation to stereotyped rules, not modulated by the context. Typical statements are the following: "I may be wrong, but I always try to be coherent," "I find it very difficult to change my mind about something," "I feel very responsible for my social duties," "When I do something, I often wonder what others expect from me."

Typically heteronomia consists in an unconditional obedience to pre-established and socially recognized *roles* (see above). Identity arises in social experience, possesses a social structure, and is best thought of as a process. The development of one's identity is dependent on learning to take the role of the other. Role taking requires imagining how personal behavior will be regarded from the standpoint of others. Roles are external representatives of identity. Roll identity is that which each person adopts on the basis of her own social function. Ego-identity goes beyond simple and straightforward identification with one's role. Role-distance is necessary to preserve the dialectic between roll identity and self-identity, that is, the dialectic between self-continuity/coherence and adaptation to new situations (Kraus, 1987). Roll identity is to TMs not a part of the dialectic process necessary for establishing one's self-identity. Rather, it is a shelter to protect their own fragile self-identity. The role is a sort of external crutch, an *exoskeleton*, which supports a crippled self-identity. This dialectic is absent in TMs, as they are unable to go beyond socially established roles, to modify their own social role and attune it to the manifold of existential circumstances.

Intolerance of Ambiguity

Intolerance of ambiguity is the inability to accommodate and anticipate the coexistence of opposite characteristics in an object, person, or relationship. We described the

Table 15.2 Values in *typus melancholicus* (TM)

Values

1. Conscientiousness: commitment to prevent guilt attributions and guilt feelings; effort to feel accepted by others.

2. Orderliness: fixation on harmony in interpersonal relationships (need to avoid conflicts).

3. Hyper/heteronomia: exaggerated norm adaptation (hypernomia) and norm receptiveness (heteronomia).

4. Intolerance of ambiguity: inability to accommodate and anticipate the coexistence of opposite characteristics in an object, person, or relationship.

emotional side of this characteristic of TMs earlier. The negative emotion provoked by the perception of contradictory features in one person or situation crystallizes in a value, a kind of moral Manichaeism. Emotional intolerance of ambiguity, that is, proneness to develop negative emotions if in the presence of ambiguity, develops into a special kind of intolerance or ego-syntonic narrow-mindedness. One's incapacity to appreciate complexity develops into a blaming attitude towards the complexity and ambiguity that is intrinsic to the *condició humana*. Typical statements are "I need to be reassured about the qualities of the persons around me," "If something shakes my certainties, I can easily get into a crisis," "I felt as if I were paralyzed when I realized that she/he was not the honest person I had thought before," "I feel very bad when someone whom I like behaves in an unexpected way to me."

The need to include oneself within a rigid identity makes it necessary to see others reduced to a generic prototype. Intolerance of ambiguity permits the TM to only experience social situations that confirm the pre-established image they have of themselves and of others. This compromises the capacity of maintaining true interpersonal relationships and contemplating situations that presuppose recognition of emotive complexity. The TM is not capable of perceiving their own individuality and that of others (idioagnosia), given that the exemplary prototype completely absorbs their attention. In this sense, their intersubjectivity is mutilated (pseudo-intersubjectivity), while deprived of the emotive implications regarding recognition of one's own subjectivity and that of the other. In fact, relating with the Other only through their role, the TM does not respond to needs, desires, and individual feelings. The TM only responds to that which is directly derivable from the social identity. Their altruistic availability is not directed at the other as an *individuum*, but rather is aimed at maintaining social balance based on the effort of synchronizing with the Other according to predetermined rules and roles.

Table 15.2 summarizes the values of persons with *typus melancholicus*.

Pre-Melancholic Limit Situation

To sum up: the TM personality is phenomenally characterized by the need for meticulous organization of one's own life-world and the fixation on harmony in interpersonal relationships; the commitment to prevent guilt attributions and guilt feelings; an exaggerated norm adaptation and external norm receptiveness; and by the emotional and cognitive incapacity to perceive opposite characteristics concerning the same object or person (Stanghellini and Bertelli, 2006).

Melancholia, as all mental disorders, occurs within the context of a pre-morbid personality structure that has a profound effect on the pathogenesis, presentation, and course of the disorder itself. In the case of TM, the notion of pre-morbid personality is intended in a specific pathogenetic sense, i.e. TM personality is a predisposing factor to the development of an episode of melancholia through a specific type of pre-melancholic limit situation. There is a relationship of complementarity between the TM pre-morbid personality and the pre-melancholic situation.

The concept of "situation" indicates a person's way of living the relationship with the world in a reciprocal exchange, a relationship of interdependence with the context, especially social context. The *habitus* of person (Stanghellini, 2016a), that is (generally speaking), her way of understanding life and expressing relationships with the Other, the hierarchy of her priorities and values, leads her to have a kind of relationship that is typical for this person. We can say that each type of person tends to constitute a given type of self–world situation. The notion of situation covers both the active role in the sense that the person actively concurs in creating the situation and the passive role in the sense that there is not an explicit or voluntary intention or desire to create that typical situation. Through her typical situation, the person is aware of her own incapacity of existing any other way (Stanghellini and Bertelli, 2006).

The kind of situation that the TM concurs to generate, namely the pre-melancholic situation, is characterized by a constant increase of the fixed tasks that overburdens the capacity of the TM to preserve a predetermined order. In such conditions, the TM is not capable of establishing a hierarchy of priorities, and is unable to discriminate what can be momentarily left aside or postponed. In this context two constellations emerge that characterize the pre-melancholic phase, namely *includence* and *remanence*, followed by the radical transformation of the self–world relation called *despair*.

Includence

Includence indicates a self-contradiction that sees the TM, at one and the same time, engaged in an extreme attempt to maintain order while needing to overcome it, exceeding the TM's own limits. This is the moment in which the undesired is manifested and imposed in the TM's existence, so that the typical meticulous and orderly form of being of the TM is destabilized. As an example, a TM person typically engages in a kind of life-project in which she ends up being overburdened by a number of commitments she is no longer able to accomplish.

Remanence

Remanence is characterized by remaining behind these commitments. The TM is conditioned by the paradoxical tendency of canceling possible debts in advance. When they are up against the unexpected and chance and unforeseen factors break into one's schemes, this may precipitate a melancholic episode.

The two constellations are always manifested in the pre-melancholic situation, but they are not clear until the melancholic phase has begun. The bridge that joins the pre-melancholic phase to the melancholic one is called despair.

Despair

The key feature of the pre-melancholic situation is despair. The concept of "despair" cannot be translated either as hopelessness or helplessness as this concept does not indicate, in fact, either loss of hope or feeling deprived of establishing the possibility of being helped. Rather, with the term despair, "coming and going" towards unreachable possibilities is indicated. Despair is a state of emotional-cognitive dissonance characterized by the incapacity to establish priorities, a situation in which one cannot make any decision.

Despair is the prodrome of melancholic breakdown. Tellenbach emphasizes the intimate relation between the concept of "despair" (*Verzweiflung*) and the notion of "doubt" (*Zweifel*) as a disintegration of something simple and definitive into something ambiguous:

> the crucial emphasis, as also in the concept of doubt [*Zweifel*], shifts to the "two," to the doubling. This doubling [*zweiheitliche*] is also contained in dubietas and dubium. What we call despair [*Verzweiflung*] is remaining captured in doubt. From the doubling of despair results all average meanings of human states characterized by being shattered [*Zerrissenheit*]. To be precise, despair is not just hopelessness and desperation, not an ultimate or an arrival at an endpoint, but rather the movement backward and forward, an alternation, so that a definite decision [*endgültige Entscheidung*] is no longer possible. (Tellenbach, 1961/1980: 165 [149]; translation modified)

As a consequence of the ambiguity, the person experiences ambivalent feelings in the sense of being simultaneously moved towards two opposite directions. The person is aware of this contradiction, but is not able to resolve it. The core of despair is therefore indecision, and its contrary mental state is not hope, but decision. In despair, this opposition comes to an extreme which results in a profound alteration of temporality: "[w]hat previously came about in the mode of succession, now appears only in the necessity of simultaneity" (Tellenbach, 1961/1980: 167 [151]). The same happens with lived space. Whereas we usually organize our actions in the mode of succession, in despair movements remain stuck in the indecisiveness of juxtaposition, that is, a kind of paralysis of action and thinking, but not a static one, rather a frenzied, restless, disconcerting paralysis.

The Life-World of Persons with Melancholia

In the following paragraphs, we continue with the description of the basic structures of the life-world within which the experience of persons affected by acute melancholic episodes is situated, including abnormal experiences of time, space, body, self and others, and their modifications. These descriptions accurately describe and make sense of psychopathological experiences, and help us to answer the question "What is it like to be melancholic?"

Lived Time

Melancholia has been conceptualized as a disorder of lived time (see Minkowski, 1933/1970; Straus, 1947; Binswanger, 1960; Tatossian, 1975; Kimura, 1992; Fuchs, 2001, 2013a, 2014; Northoff, 2016a, 2016b; Northoff and Stanghellini, 2016; Stanghellini, Ballerini, et al., 2016).

In order to understand *"what is"* and *"how happens"* the time in acute melancholic episodes, it should be recalled that there are two "moments" of pre-phenomenal time which can be designated "synthesis" and "conation" (see Chapter 6). The concept of "synthesis" describes the construction of the associative connections bridging succeeding moments of consciousness, namely past, present, and future. Conation (from Latin *conatus* = effort, drive) is the basic "energetic momentum" of mental life which contributes to self- and world-awareness with the sense of aliveness and spontaneity which may be regarded as the essence of subjective life (Fuchs, 2013a). This kind of movement is embedded in the social relationships to others, indeed we move forward into a promising future because we feel co-temporal with other persons (Fuchs, 2013a).

Melancholic symptoms have been conceptualized as connected to a crisis of conation. With a standstill of becoming, the future is rendered inaccessible. The past cannot be dissipated, but lies heavy and over-determining. Discordance between subjective and objective time is experienced as the vanishing of time (existence does not grow in the stream of time) accompanied by a sense of unreality since the feeling of "reality" is based on the synchronization and coexistence of the world and one's own self. Persons affected by melancholia do not feel equal to the speed of external changes or to necessary developments. They refrain from necessary role changes and shrink from confrontation with the basic facts of existence such as isolation, finiteness, decision, and guilt and fail in achieving forgetting and elimination of the past. Normally, the past withdraws from one's field of experience as the future appears as a space open to movement and change. Absence of temporal movement may generate a view of the future that appears static, deterministic, and hopeless.

We identify three categories of disorders of lived time in acute melancholia (Stanghellini, Ballerini, et al., 2016):

(1) Vital retardation

This category responds to the question: "How do patients experience their body as related to temporal becoming?" Patients experience a stagnation of bodily functions and the exhaustion of their body as the source of vitality and becoming. Their bodily functions are slowed down or blocked; their organs are emptied, imploded, or putrefied. Typical sentences are: "I can't eat or drink because the bowel is blocked"; "Body not working, drained of energy"; "Stomach fallen down, seed or wheat germ are stuck in gullet"; "I have no eyes, I have no face, they are gone, no back passage, no body, no hands."

(2) Present and future dominated by the past

This category responds to the question: "Are patients more focused on the present, past, or future?" Patients are preoccupied with past events and less focused on future or present ones. Patients' temporal experience is overwhelmed by the impact of the past: the "already spent" prevails. The past is experienced as irrevocably established, the present and the future as a repetition of the past. Typical sentences are: "Future gloomy, invaded by the past"; "Sometimes I didn't know what to do with the wreck I was"; "Guilt about past life suffocates me"; "I'm guilty of many things in the past"; "I have to be punished for past misdeeds"; "I'm terrified because I have done something in the past."

(3) Slackening of the flow of time

This category responds to the question: "How do patients experience the flow of time?" Patients experience an inhibition of becoming. The present moment does not flow in the direction of the future. This category includes two subcategories:

(a) Slowing down of the flow of time

Patients live the flow of time as slowed down. It is a time that drags. Patients feel that the present moment is dilated. Typical sentence are: "Very long day and long night"; "I'm dying slowly"; "Time seemed an eternity"; "Time seems to drag"; "Time slowed down"; "I speak slowly."

(b) Blocking of the flow of time

Patients live time as a stagnating standstill. It is a time that does not develop anymore. Patients feel that the present moment is frozen. Whereas in the slowing down of the flow of time subcategory the main characteristic is that the present is expanded, here the world may be experienced as if no new meaningful events can occur, or as if one's identity cannot be further modified. Typical sentences are: "Time is void"; "I can't remember days because time is stopped"; "I lost the flow of time"; "I dread organizing things because time came to a stop"; "Time is hopeless"; "I can never repeat the circumstance of the present time."

Lived Body

The essential, substantive feature of melancholia is a change in finding oneself in one's own body, that is to say, in a modification of the lived that basically consists in a commitment of "vital feelings," in Scheler's sense (1973) (see Schneider, 1935; López-Ibor, 1974; Dörr-Zegers and Tellenbach, 1980; Dörr-Zegers, 1993). The radical alteration has to be found in the world of vitality, of basic needs, drives, and emotions; ultimately, of vital feelings (Dörr-Zeghers and Stanghellini, 2015). "My body is dead"; "My interiority is lifeless"; "I feel deprived of all sorts of sparkle coming from within"; "I cannot feel"; "I cannot be impressed by what's going on around me"; "I don't feel empty, I am empty" – these are just a few examples of the lived corporeality of persons with depression. It is a feeling of diminished vitality, freshness, physical and psychical integrity that dominates the existence of melancholics.

The body I am has at least two aspects: the body-as-support and the body-as-willing (Zutt, 1963). The first aspect, the *tragender Leib* (body-as-support) in Zutt's psychiatric anthropology, corresponds to the vital region called "affective-vegetative." It is constituted by the involuntary and pre-reflexive background of our needs (e.g. hunger, thirst, sleepiness, sexual desire) and vital feelings (e.g. courage/discouragement, vitality/fatigue, pleasure/nausea, etc.). Needs and vital feelings direct us to the world and to the objects of interest that populate it. The body-as-support is the seat of autonomous processes (moods and drives) that move us/stop us. This dimension of the lived body is characterized as being in greater or lesser measure alien to the will (I cannot decide to be hungry or sleepy or euphoric or tired) and subject to the time of maturation, of becoming, also certainly involuntary.

The lived body in persons with depression reflects sinking, loss of support, and loss of being carried – all dimensions of the body-as-support. The modification of corporeality, observed by looking at a person affected by melancholia, reflects a disorder of this dimension, as shown by these patients' complaints: discouragement, lack of energy, lack of strength, heaviness of limbs, feeling of cold, nausea, generalized pain, etc.

In melancholia, the body, which usually represents the flexible medium through which we have contact with our world, acts as an obstacle between the self and the world. Persons affected by melancholia are confined within a body that has lost its fluidity, mobility, and flexibility, having become, instead, solid and heavy; it resists any attempt at reaching out to touch the external world. The body, just like space and time, sinks into itself, into its own geometrical confines. It loses the lightness, fluidity, and mobility of a medium and turns into a heavy, solid body which puts up resistance to all intentions and impulses directed towards the world. In melancholia, the lived body, which used to connect oneself with the world and with other people, closes itself up, thus taking on the aspect of a corpse. Dörr-Zegers (1995) talks about this in terms of a "chrematic transformation" (*chrema* = corpse) of the body as the turning point of an early feeling of melancholia. *Chrema* is the inanimate nature to which the melancholic's body is reduced, losing its enclave in the world.

Melancholic patients experience an oppression and constriction that may focus on single areas of the body – for example, feeling armor or a tire around the chest, of a lump in the throat, pressure in the head – or also manifested in a diffuse anxiety, an overall bodily rigidity. The fluid body coagulates either into a single part of itself, or into an organ, which is then felt to be heavy, weighty, oppressive, and suffocating. The materiality, density, and weight of the body, otherwise suspended and unnoticed in everyday performance, now come to the forefront and are felt painfully.

In this respect, melancholia closely resembles somatic illnesses such as infections that affect one's overall bodily state. Corresponding reports from patients may well be elicited provided that the interviewer takes their bodily experience seriously: they will complain about feelings of fatigue, exhaustion, paralysis, aches, sickness, nausea, numbness, etc. Yet there is a fundamental difference between the experience of pain and exhaustion that we find in melancholia compared to that we may find in somatic illness: in the former there is an over-identification with one's sick body that is not present in the latter. We often say "fall into depression," by which we mean that one is falling into something other than one's self, just as if one were sinking into a hole in the ground; instead, what's really happening in melancholia is that one is falling into oneself. The overall structure of this experience of depersonalization can be better understood if we widen our approach to include a fundamental aspect of the melancholic existence: the phenomenon of centricity, or over-identification. An important and distinctive feature of embodiment in persons with melancholia is its being dominated by the structure of over-identification in the sense of Kraus (1977, 1995). These patients can feel that they are nothing but their body which is experienced as abnormally materialized and reified, heavy and rigid, devoid of emotions, energies, and drives.

This loss of bodily elasticity and resonance implies painful sensations of derealization (feelings of detachment from other persons and external reality). In melancholia the exchange of body and environment is blocked, and drive and impulse are exhausted. The constriction and encapsulation of the body corresponds to the psychosocial experiences that typically lead to depression. These are experiences of a disruption of relations and bonds, including the loss of relevant others or of important social roles, further situations of a backlog in one's duties, falling short of one's aspirations, or social defeat. These situations of social separation or defeat are perceived as particularly threatening since the patients feel they do not have the necessary resources for coping ("learned helplessness"). Melancholia can be understood as the consequent psychophysiological reaction: on the biological level, it involves a pattern of neurobiological, metabolic, immunological, biorhythmic, and other organismic dysfunctions which are equivalent to a partial decoupling or separation between organism and environment. These dysfunctions are subjectively experienced as a loss of drive and interest (anhedonia), psychomotor inhibition, bodily constriction, and depressive mood.

Lived Space

The physiognomy of space in melancholia is strictly related with the way patients experience both time and their body. They experience a sense of bodily constriction which expresses a special kind of anxiety, namely anguish. Concomitant with this sense of bodily constriction there is a metamorphosis of lived distance between oneself and things in the world which may be experienced as out of reach and inaccessible (Straus, 1958).

Constriction continues in sensorimotor space: patients are not able to vividly participate in the environment, their gaze gets tired and empty, their interest weakens. Stagnation in this domain consists in the fact that melancholic patients are only able to passively receive what comes from outside. In order to act, patients have to overcome the inhibition and, indeed, the external aims and objects withdraw from the patient. In Heidegger's terms, things in the world are not "ready-to-hand," but simply "there" (*zuhanden* vs. *vorhanden*) (Fuchs, 2005, 2014). In other words, there is a growth of distance between one's body and the outside world, in concomitance with one's body constriction and inhibition and the blocking of lived time, that culminate in depressive stupor.

Self

Melancholia does not entail disorders of the pre-reflexive self as is the case with schizophrenia. It implies a different kind of depersonalization involving the process through which we form the representation of our identity, that is, the narrative self. The narrative self is the concept one constructs of oneself. One's own narrative identity arises from the interplay between I-am's and I-can's. I-can's are what one is not, one's own possibilities. Melancholics insist on a finite and unchosen perspective of stable characteristics that they consider their own, and with which they over-identify and experience other possibilities merely as a source of alienation or nullification (Kraus, 1977, 1991, 1996) This intolerance to other possibilities and the avoidance of the dialectic between I-am's and I-can's in the constitution of one's narrative self leads to an identification with partial, external, and reified identities, such as roll identity, i.e. external/socially appreciated representations of identity (Mundt et al.,1996; Stanghellini and Bertelli, 2006).

The internalized roll identities of oneself and of others are jeopardized during the premelancholic limit situation and finally break down during acute melancholic episodes. Painful feelings of depersonalization arise before one's identity is menaced by the excruciating certainty of having lost one's moral, physical, and financial integrity. Persons affected by melancholia experience themselves as guilty of not being able to love other people and to feel compassion for them.

Otherness

The loss of bodily resonance or affectability concerns, more generally, the experience of affective valences and atmospheres. The deeper the melancholia, the more the attractive qualities of the environment fade. The patients are no longer capable of being moved and affected by things, situations, or other persons. This leads to an inability to feel emotions or atmospheres at all, which is all the more painful as it is not caused by mere apathy or indifference, but by the tormenting bodily constriction and rigidity. Kurt Schneider (1920) wrote that the "vital disturbances" of bodily feelings in severe depression are so intense that psychic or "higher" feelings can no longer arise. This does not seem to be entirely correct: this profound indifference to others is experienced as a source of suffering. Complaints of loss of emotional resonance (e.g. the incapacity to have empathic feelings for others) are typical in acute episodes. Another distinctive feature is that these experiences have the paradoxical character of a painful lack of feeling, an excruciating incapacity to be affected,

Table 15.3 The life-world of persons with melancholia

Existential	Experiences
Time	Crisis of conation
	Discordance between subjective and objective time
	Vanishing of time accompanied by a sense of unreality
	Vital retardation
	Present and future dominated by the past
	Slackening of the flow of time
Space	Experience of bodily constriction
	Constriction continues in sensorimotor space
	Metamorphosis of lived distance between oneself and things in the world which may be experienced as inaccessible
	Growth of distance between one's body and the outside world, in concomitance with one's body constriction
Body	Diminished vital feelings
	The body (which usually represents the flexible medium with which we have contact with our world) acts as an obstacle between the self and the world
	It turns into a heavy, solid body which puts up resistance to all intentions and impulses directed towards the world
Other	The other is over-identified with its social role
	Complaints of loss of emotional resonance
	Ethic depersonalization
Self	Suspension of "being-with"
	Interruption of the dialectic between I-am's and I-can's. This involves an identification with partial, external, and reified identities, such as roll identity, i.e. external/socially appreciated representations of identity
	Excruciating certainty of having lost one's moral, physical, and financial integrity

the feeling of the loss of feelings – quite the opposite of ataraxia. In fact, melancholic patients stigmatize their emotional anaesthesia; their overall attitude towards this phenomenon is, first of all, and for the most part, characterized by self-accusing, self-reprimanding, and a sense of guilt. Also, due to their psychomotor inhibition they feel a burden to others since they are not able to be self-sufficient. Persons affected by melancholia especially stigmatize their own inability to love, and push themselves to repudiate the inauthenticity of their own previous over-involvement with the others, i.e. the kind of feelings they used to have when free of melancholic acute states. This is known as "the motive of the lie in melancholics" (Kraus, 1995). It highlights how the melancholic depersonalization is an ethic depersonalization: rarely does the melancholic limit herself to merely acknowledging the loss of ability to love, rather her whole experience is permeated by her judgments on what is right or wrong, authentic or inauthentic, sincere or dishonest, and by the anguishing doubt about which of the two selves – the current or the preceding one – is the real one, without faking. All this leads to a radical solitude and to a suspension of "being-with."

Table 15.3 summarizes the life-world of persons with melancholia.

The Life-World of Persons with Feeding and Eating Disorders

Introduction

Feeding and eating disorders (FED) encompass three main diagnoses: anorexia nervosa, bulimia nervosa, and binge eating disorder. However, the collection of disturbances of eating attitudes and behaviors includes several other conditions such as pica, rumination disorder, purging disorder, atypical anorexia and bulimia nervosa, subthreshold binge eating disorder, and night eating syndrome. Longitudinal studies indicate that most patients migrate among diagnoses over time (Fairburn, Cooper, and Shafran, 2003; Milos et al., 2005) without a substantial change in basic psychopathological features (Tozzi et al., 2005; Fairburn and Cooper, 2007; Eddy et al., 2008) suggesting the existence of a common psychopathological core.

All these conditions display key similarities that can be divided into two main psychopathological domains: behavioral and experiential disorders. Behavioral anomalies include binge eating, dietary restraint, compensatory purging, and body checking. Abnormal experiences include preoccupations with one's weight and shape and an anomalous perception of these. There is a general agreement on considering behavioral anomalies – which are required for DSM diagnosis – as secondary epiphenomena to a more basic psychopathological core, namely excessive concerns about body shape and weight.

Furthermore, these concerns have been associated with a more profound disturbance consisting in disorders of the way persons experience their own body. At the core of FED there is a disorder of the lived body. Persons prone to FED often report – with different extents of insight – their difficulties in perceiving their emotions and that they do not "feel" themselves. They have difficulties in feeling their own body in the first-person perspective and in having a stable and continuous sense of themselves as embodied agents. What they seem to lack is the coenesthetic apprehension of their own body as the more primitive and basic form of self-awareness.

The disturbance of the experience of their own body is interconnected with the process of shaping their personal identity. Indeed, we construe our personal identity on the basis of our feelings, that is, of what we like or dislike. We appraise the value of things in the world through our body as we feel attracted or indifferent to them. This is the way we understand who we are and what we want to be. Difficulties in feeling oneself reflect difficulties in perceiving one's emotions. Indeed, feeling oneself is a basic requirement for achieving an identity and a stable sense of one's self (Stanghellini, Trisolini, et al., 2014). The experience of not feeling one's own body and emotions involves the whole sense of identity. If a person can hardly feel herself and her feelings are discontinuous over time, her identity is no longer a real psychic structure that persists beyond the flow of time and circumstances. This person will also feel extraneous from her own body and attempts to regain a sense of bodily self through coping strategies like starvation or quantification:

PATIENT: "I will ask my GP to prescribe me some blood tests. I need numbers."

THERAPIST: "Why?"

PATIENT: *"To be scared."*

THERAPIST: "Why do you need numbers to get scared?"

PATIENT: "Because I do not trust what I feel in my body."

Bodily experience and the shaping and construction of identity are interconnected. Therefore, abnormal bodily experiences and attitudes towards one's own corporeality, and related difficulties in the definition of one's own identity, have been proposed as the core features of FED (Stanghellini, Castellini, et al., 2012; Stanghellini, Trisolini, et al., 2014; Castellini et al., 2015, 2017; Stanghellini, Mancini, et al., forthcoming). Whereas most people evaluate and define themselves on the basis of the way they feel in various situations and perceive their performance in various domains, patients with FED judge their self-worth largely, or even exclusively, in terms of their shape and weight and their ability to control them.

"Having my weight under control makes me feel in control of my emotional states"; "If my measurements remain the same over time I feel that I am myself, if not I feel I am getting lost."

"I believe in bathroom scales as an indicator of my daily successes and failures."
(*Source*: theproanalifestyleforever [blog])

In this chapter, we develop the idea that persons who overvalue their body shape and weight can be better understood as suffering from a specific disorder of lived corporeality, and more specifically as the predominance of one dimension of embodiment, namely the "lived-body-for-others." Persons with FED experience their own body first and foremost as an object being looked at by another, rather than coenesthetically or from a first-person perspective. Alienation from one's own body and from one's own emotions, disgust for it, shame, and an exaggerated concern to take responsibility for the way one appears to others, as well as the need to feel oneself only through the gaze of the others, through objective measures and through self-starvation, i.e. many of the features of persons with FED, can be illuminated by looking at it in the light of the Sartrean concept of feeling a "lived-body-for-others" (Sartre, 1943/1992).

The Lived-Body-for-Others

In Chapter 6 we explained the distinction between body-subject and body-object. The first is the body experienced from within, my own direct experience of my body in the first-person perspective, myself as a spatiotemporal embodied agent in the world; the second is the body thematically investigated from without, as for example by natural sciences such as anatomy and physiology, a third-person perspective (Husserl, 1912–1915; Merleau-Ponty, 1945/1962). One's own body can be apprehended by a person in the first-person perspective as the body-I-am. This is the coenesthetic apprehension of one's own body, the primitive experience of oneself, the direct, unmediated experience of one's own facticity, including oneself as *this* body, its form, height, weight, color, as well as one's past and what is actually happening. First and foremost, we have an implicit acquaintance with our own body from the first-person perspective. The lived body turns into a physical, objective body whenever we become aware of it in a disturbing way. Whenever our movement is somehow impeded or disrupted, the lived body is thrown back on itself, materialized or "corporealized." It becomes an object for me. Having been a living bodily being before, I now realize that I have a material (impeding, clumsy, vulnerable, finite, etc.) body (Fuchs, 2002).

In addition to these two dimensions of corporeality, Sartre (1943/1992) emphasized that one can apprehend one's own body also from another vantage point, as one's own body *when it is looked at by another person.* When I become aware that I, or better that my own body is looked at by another person, I realize that my body can be an object for that person. Sartre calls this the "lived-body-for-others." "With the appearance of the Other's look," writes Sartre, "I experience the revelation of my being-as-object." The upshot of this is a feeling of "having my being outside . . . [the feeling] of being an object" (Sartre, 1943/1992: 351–352). Thus, one's identity becomes reified by the gaze of the Other, and reduced to the external appearance of one's own body.

One of us (Stanghellini, 2016a) reported the paradigmatic case study of a young girl who experiences her own body first and foremost as an object being looked at by another, rather than from a first-person perspective. Since she cannot have an experience of her body from within, she apprehends her body from without through the gaze of the Other. Her body is to her as a "wobbling liquid" which may change when she is in the presence of other persons. Her body, so to say, takes the shape that the Other's gaze imposes upon it. This is the source of her exaggerated concern to take responsibility for the way she appears to Others. The Other's gaze makes her feel shame or disgust for her body. This is why she first and foremost avoids contact with other persons.

Yet, it is not always shame and alienation from her body that take place when she is looked at by other persons. At sunset, protected by semi-obscurity, she strolls in front of a bar crowded with young people. Being the object of their gazes she can finally feel herself as a body being looked at. The Other's gaze helps her recover a sense of "unity" and "condensation." "The way I feel depends on the way I feel looked at by the others" and "Sometimes I focalize myself through the gaze of the others" are typical sentences by persons affected by FED. Other typical sentences are "Knowing what the others think of me calms me down," "I can't stand not to know what the others think of me," "For me it's very important to see myself through the eyes of the others," "When I meet someone I can't stay without knowing what he thinks of me," "I am dependent on the evaluation of the others," "Even if I think that the way the others evaluate me is wrong, I can't do without it" (quotes from Stanghellini, Castellini, et al., 2012).

The body shapes identity and the way that we form and participate within social relationships. For FED persons causality seems to go in the opposite direction: social relationships shape identity. Yet it may be difficult to go this way to get acquainted with oneself as the Other's gaze may not be unequivocal:

"What is your image?"

"I wish I knew!! It can be so hard to tell what others think of you."

The Other

FED patients define themselves by the gaze of other persons. The way they feel, even the very possibility to feel themselves, depends on the way they feel looked at by others.

In the life-world of these persons the Other is reduced to its gaze. The Other's look only seizes what is visible, that is, appearance. Also, it only seizes what is present here and now. The temporal dimension of the gaze is the present moment. The gaze does not even expand into the nearest future, as it might in the case of someone gazing at someone else while the latter replies with her own gaze. There is not a dialogue of gazes. The Other is not a partner with whom one can dialogue.

Why I starve myself?

Because of all the people in my life who die of jealousy when they see the way I look
(*Source*: thepronalifestyleforever)

What does the Other's gaze express? It can simply express like or dislike, recognition or non-recognition. The Other is a gaze and the patient is a body looking for visual recognition. The Other is a gaze that may (or may not) like her. Feeling liked or non-liked helps recover a sense of selfhood and identity, at least in the aesthetic dimension as a here-and-now body object of the Other's desire. The Other is hardly an interlocutor with whom to engage an intersubjective co-creativity relationship. He is the one who confirms my existence, my being-in-the-world. The gaze of the Other becomes the unique way through which one can be aware of one's own presence. It is the mirror in which to see oneself and feel oneself.

In this perspective, the life-world of persons with FED reflects the essential features of late modernity (Stanghellini, 2005): the experience of persons who feel they exist only through the eyes of the others. Only what is visible exists. What we can't see doesn't exist. If no one can see what you have done, what you have done does not exist. The feeling of being a Self and having an identity can be so weak that one may feel one becomes real only when one is *the topic of a discourse*. Someone who is not relating to some other is in a liquid state; when faced with the Other one becomes semi-solid, but at the expense of getting the form imposed by the gaze and the discourse of the Other. Only being seen or being talked about gives substance to the Self. Being seen and being talked about by others take the place of the self-feeling of oneself. These are the answers taken from a ProAna[1] blog entitled "*I will finally feel skinny when . . .*":

"When I'm the 'skinny friend'."

"When people ask me if I've lost weight."

Ours is an age of pure relationality, on condition that we remove all moral overtones from this word. Pure relationality is self-referencing. The Other is a means, the mirror through which I can apprehend myself. No true dialectic exists between oneself and the Other. The Self takes on the Other's shape, or the shape of that which the Self believes are the Other's expectations – or stubbornly tries to resist the shape the Other wants to impose upon

---

[1] ProAna organizations differ widely in their stances. Most claim that they exist mainly as a non-judgmental environment for persons with anorexia, others deny anorexia nervosa is a mental illness and claim instead that it is a "lifestyle choice" that should be respected.

oneself. The relationship with the Other is an instrumental one, aimed at obtaining a view on oneself. This is also the case with one's relation with one's own body. In the age of the "industrialization of the body" (Rilke, 1910/1990), we are not our own body, rather *we use it*. The body is not the silent background from which one's own sense of selfhood and personal identity develops, but a subject of choice. The body is a task. There is a total symmetry between controlling and shaping one's body and controlling and shaping one's life. The body is a fetish taking the place of identity: body-building takes the place of the *Bildung* of oneself as a person

Selfhood and Identity

There is a general agreement to consider the maintenance of FED as based on a dysfunctional system for evaluating self-worth. Whereas most people evaluate themselves on the basis of their perceived performance in a variety of domains of life (e.g. the quality of their relationships, work, parenting, sporting ability, etc.), people with FED judge themselves largely, or even exclusively, in terms of their eating habits, shape, or weight and their ability to control them.

The relevance of feeding for the development of basic forms of selfhood is quite evident. Feeding represents a vital activity for the construction of the Self since it serves as a framing environment and allows face-to-face contact with the caregiver via the phenomenon of affective attunement (Stern, 1985/2000). Also, the experience of one's own body is interconnected with the process of shaping one's personal identity. The coenesthetic apprehension of one's own body is the more primitive and basic form of self-awareness or core Self. Indeed, feeling oneself is a basic requirement to achieve a stable sense of one's Self and the basic condition of possibility for developing a narrative apprehension of oneself or autobiographical Self.

Patients with FED often report their difficulties in feeling themselves, especially their own body, and in perceiving their emotions: "Sometimes, the emotions I feel are extraneous to me and scare me"; "I see myself out of focus, I don't feel myself." The experience of not feeling one's own body and emotions involves the whole sense of identity. For persons prone to FED, the identity is no longer a real psychic structure that persists beyond the flow of time and circumstances.

Therefore, there is the need to resort to one's own body weight as a viable source of definition of the Self. Anorectic persons may explain their behavior as a tool for achieving a new identity (Nordbø, 2006) since changing one's body is a tool to become another (Skarderud, 2007a, 2007b). They want to change, and changing one's body serves as a concrete and symbolic tool for such ambition. Thus, shaping oneself is a "concretized metaphor," establishing equivalence between a psychic reality (identity) and a physical one (one's body shape).

To persons affected by FED identity is a task, not a taken-for-granted datum. They have the necessity to perpetually construct themselves. This construction is based on the way they feel seen and judged by other persons. In this perspective, they seem to share with the late-modern mind an aesthetic or *pornographic* conceptualization of the Self based on seeing and been seen and on the approval of others.

"I will finally feel skinny when . . .":

"When I'm no longer embarrassed to take pictures/be in pictures."

"When people start calling me the girl who is anorexic behind my back as opposed to the girl who was anorexic."

"When my parents call an intervention."

"When people are worried about my health cause I'm too thin."

In the latter case it the disapproval of others that is the measure of success and hospitalization feels like an achievement.

Another feature that FED people share with the *Zeitgeist* is the obsession with measures and numbers. Ironically, we assist in a sort of operationalization of the process of establishing one's own identity.

"I will finally feel skinny when . . .":

"When the number on the scale is my goal weight."

"No excuses, just the number."

"Recently, and I'm not even sure how it happened, I have become so neurotic about only weighing myself at the 'perfect' time."

To sum up: most pathological eating behaviors and features are a consequence of the severity of an abnormal experience of one's body and identity disorders. Persons affected by FED have difficulties in feeling their own body and emotions and try to cope with this by feeling themselves through the gaze of the Other and defining themselves through the evaluation of the Other. Other ways to cope with their basic feeling of extraneousness from their bodily self are feeling oneself through objective measures, e.g. weight and size, as well as through starvation, physical activity, and fatigue.

Each of these domains shows a typical pattern of association with the symptomatological features of patients reporting anorexia nervosa, bulimia nervosa, and binge eating disorder. Feeling oneself through the gaze of the Other and defining oneself through the evaluation of the Other are associated with overvalued thoughts regarding body shape. Alienation from one's own body and emotions, and feeling extraneous from one's own body significantly correlate with concerns about weight and body shape. Feeling oneself through objective measures and feeling oneself through starvation are associated with overvalued thoughts regarding weight and eating concerns and with dietary restriction, respectively.

Moreover, abnormal bodily experiences were observed not just for "over-threshold" FED patients, but also in subjects without full-blown FED but with abnormal eating patterns. Also, they help discriminate clinical vs. non-clinical populations. In people who develop clinically relevant FED, extraneousness from one's own body is a phenomenon that is significantly more manifest and penetrant than in people who display over-threshold, but non-full-blown abnormal eating patterns. This suggests that abnormal bodily experiences could represent a vulnerability trait in people prone to develop full-blown FED.

Time

Patients with FED report the feeling that their body can change continuously. Obviously, all human beings are affected by a dynamic person–situation interaction that involves fluid changes in the experience of one's own body. For example, there can be activating contexts such as at a party. Persons' beliefs entail self-evaluative social comparisons in which being placed within a body has ceased to be a guarantee of identity or stability, and has become a *task*.

The behavioral consequences include attempts to conceal one's body shape by covering it or restriction of social interactions. Understanding this dynamic interplay of the person and contextual events is crucial for the appreciation of body experience fluidity in everyday life. Yet the way FED people experience changes in their lived body largely exceeds the standard fluid and dynamic person–situation interaction.

These continuous fluctuations of the lived body imply the need for monitoring and controlling one's own body over time. Lived time can be reduced to a mere monitoring/control function, in particular in control and/or loss of control of weight and eating:

> "I spend most of the time in front of the mirror to control my body."

> "The perception of time depends on body control. My body is under control all the time. I fail, at times, miserably and at times I am successful, but I would like to be successful all the time."

> "One morning I feel my thighs fit perfectly in my pants, another morning instead they have become huge."

Clinicians should be aware of the situational variations of body experiences and their connection with time experience in persons with FED. Time appears to be subjectively perceived in a different way by persons with FED. For example, considering some patients with bulimia nervosa, binge eating episodes occur in a very short period of time as a breakdown in a context of continuous control of eating habits. The purging behavior occurs as a way to regain control. For both bulimia nervosa and binge eating patients, it is clear that the subjective perception of time during binge eating episodes is completely different compared with a normal time course. Patients often do not remember what they were doing, how long the episode lasted, or even what they have eaten.

An approach that overcomes merely behavioral assessment is necessary as demonstrated by the difficulties in the attempt to operationalize the definition of binge eating with objective variables like number and length of episodes or amount of food (Castellini, Trisolini, and Ricca, 2014). The consumption of a large amount of food (an amount of food that is definitely larger than most people would eat during a similar period of time and under similar circumstances) or the temporal boundary to the episode (eating in a discrete period of time, e.g. within any two-hour period), have been deeply challenged from an empirical point of view (Wolfe et al., 2009). Subjective binge eating (involving the same sense of loss of control but the consumption of a small to moderate amount of food) has been found to better predict the outcome of psychological treatments compared with objective episodes (Mond et al., 2010; Ricca et al., 2010). Also, the persistence of subjective loss of control over eating – an effect that is probably underestimated by clinicians – may contribute to relapse, by decreasing self-efficacy and confidence in maintaining the changes achieved during treatment. This kind of observation highlights the importance of adopting an experiential stance to assess and understand abnormal eating behaviors. A person's definition of a "large amount" of food as well as a "discrete period of time" is highly subjective and can be influenced by personal beliefs and rules, which can vary from day to day.

The subjective perception of time in persons with FED appears to be interconnected with the construct of control. Time is perceived in different ways on the basis of the interchange of control/loss of control phases. From an experiential point of view, the main dimension of a binge for all clinical FED conditions is based on a subjective experience of lack of control. This means that the episode exists on the basis of what a person thinks constitutes being in control. Persons with FED feel a pervasive lack of control most of the time, which results in a continuous and strong resistance against an imminent threat. This can be related to the feeling that their body can change continuously. As we said earlier, being placed within a body has ceased to be a guarantee of identity or stability, and has become a *task*. Thus, they commonly restrict their experience and focus on eating and body size to regain a feeling of control and achieve some degree of predictability in their life (Williams, Chamove, and Millar, 1990; Sassaroli, Gallucci, and Ruggiero, 2008).

Emotions: Anorexia as Passion

The emotional life of persons with FED is characterized by feelings of depersonalization. They feel extraneous from their body and emotions and this experience of not feeling oneself involves their whole sense of identity. This kind of emotional depersonalization is different from the one occurring in melancholic persons (see Chapter 15) since the latter suffer from a painful feeling of being unable to feel. Melancholic persons are deeply concerned with their incapacity to feel, and feel guilty for that. Their specific concern is *loss*, since what they fear is, next to the horror of losing one's capacity to feel, losing one's innocence (guilt), physical integrity (illness), and financial integrity (ruin).

Also, the kind of emotional depersonalization in persons with FED is different from depersonalization in persons with schizophrenia since in persons with FED we do not find the schizoid emotional ataxia we described in Chapter 14. Also disorders of enactment, engagement, and attunement are not typical. Last but not least, perplexity in the sense of *trema* is extremely uncommon: FED persons do not live in an unfamiliar and uncanny world where the capacity to maintain a relationship with oneself and the world is threatened. This kind of ontological insecurity or vulnerability is more basic than shame, guilt, or sense of social inferiority: it is the sense that one's very self is unstable and vulnerable to imploding or to being destroyed or annihilated by others.

Some analogies between the emotional life of FED and borderline persons (see Chapter 13) can be drawn, as for instance they can both experience deep feelings of shame, but FED patients do not display the typical dysphoria–anger oscillations characterizing borderline persons. Also, borderline persons typically feel unquiet about their own body, but their concern is basically about their body as a locus of agency, that is, about what causes their body to behave in that given way (e.g. impulsively). Both borderline and FED persons may feel that their body is unable to feel, but the difference between the two is in the way they cope with this: borderline persons typically use strategies like self-harm, drugs, or promiscuity, whereas the kinds of coping strategy with respect to their emotional difficulties displayed by persons with FED (different in kind from all the other groups of patients) involve feeling oneself through the gaze of the Other and defining oneself through the evaluation of the Other, starvation, and quantification of one's body measures. These are the typical coping responses to the sense of alienation from oneself and fleeting selfhood and identity.

Next to this overall condition of emotional depersonalization, FED persons also show three specific emotions, namely disgust, shame, and anxiety. These emotions are all related to one's body: shame and disgust for the shapelessness of one's body, and anxiety related to the feeling of loss of control over the incessant changes in body shape and functions. In this chapter, we will not go into the details of shame and disgust that we discussed in the chapters dedicated to the analyses of the life-worlds of contamination obsession and of the borderline type of existence. We will confine ourselves to the specific character of these emotions in the life-world of people with FED.

As we have seen in Chapter 7, disgust is the emotion that accompanies the separation of a part from the whole. All the parts coming from the disintegration of things become waste. Anything is disgusting when it loses the harmony of completeness. We are disgusted by the physiognomy of decay, whose central characteristic is the *aneidos* or the un-form. Seemingly, discontinuity over time of body perception can contribute to the emotion of disgust towards one's own body in persons with FED, but first and foremost it is the feeling that one's "lower" bodily needs must be separated from and opposed to the "higher" spiritual values that contributes to it.

Shame seems to share this origin with disgust in persons with FED. Shame is the emotion whereby I am aware of being seen by another person whose devaluating gaze and annihilating contempt uncovers a part of who I am, usually a part that makes me feel inadequate and dishonored. This part, in the case of FED persons is obviously their body. The origin of the feeling of shame is the feeling of a sort of imbalance and disharmony between the claim of spiritual personhood and embodied needs. Shame arises by way of the contiguity between higher levels of consciousness and lower drive-awareness. Disgust and shame for one's body are rooted in one's experience of one's own bodily values as uncoupled from one's spiritual values.

Next to this feeling of shame that is related to the human condition as such, another main category of shame in FED persons refers to a general sense of being unworthy: the shame of being the person one is. This nuance of shame is closely related to guilt feelings or other "depressive" emotions like feeling insufficient, undeserving, contemptible and insignificant. Also, there are several specific or "local" intentional objects of shame (what they feel ashamed for, the focuses of their shame) in persons with FED (Skarderud, 2007a, 2007b): greed (related to food), envy (for the success of other persons), sadness (for one's own miserable condition and achievement failures), grandiosity (for challenging death through starvation), rage (against one's own fate). Other focuses of shame are one's body appearance and body function. FED persons may also feel ashamed for their lack of self-control and self-destructive behavior. Their shame can be related to sexual abuse or to experiences in which they were being made inferior. Finally, they may feel shame for suffering from FED and the related social stigma.

Shame is both a cause and consequence in FED. Shame constitutes an emotional point of departure for anorexic behavior. Individuals with negative or low self-esteem will seek ways to compensate such feelings. As we have seen, negative emotions in FED people are controlled via the concrete body. The focus of coping is on body, weight, and dietary control. Shame can also be a consequence of anorexic behavior (for instance in terms of social stigma, or failure in achieving the anorexic value of self-control), hence inducing a shame–shame cycle.

Shame is also a very relevant concept for understanding therapeutic processes. Profound shame can complicate the therapeutic process by challenging its very foundation: dialogue and the therapeutic relationship itself as health promoting. Understanding the role of shame in the therapeutic relationship can be useful for enabling therapists to persevere, by gaining an understanding of the behavior which may be experienced as a rejection (Skarderud, 2007a, 2007b).

Anxiety is a mood and as such has no specific intentional object – one single thing one can be afraid of. In anxiety one feels suspended over an inner bottomlessness, while not one single thing, but an atmosphere is felt as a menace. Narratives of persons with FED show that anxiety is the emotion that arises in them when they feel a pervasive lack of control over their body. Yet what may remain in the background is that this anxiety around food and gaining weight and the almost constant preoccupation with the control of shape and weight can be traced back to the experience of a body that has ceased to be a guarantee of selfhood and identity. Yet these feelings related to body and self mainly remain unfocused and persons with FED may be unable to make explicit the ultimate "object" from which their concern arises.

Generalizing, we can say that specific emotions like anxiety as well as disgust and shame are secondary with respect to a global feeling of emotional depersonalization. They all point to the global lack of feeling of being that lies at the bottom of the FED life-world that we must focus on in greater detail. Disgust, shame, and anxiety for one's body are deep-rooted in a special kind of feeling of incompleteness that is better understood as *shapelessness* or *lack of form*. This is not simply the lack of form in an aesthetic sense as is the case with being fat, ugly, or deformed. Rather, this feeling refers to the incapacity to give a form or shape to one's existence and to the unpredictability and uncontrollability of one's bodily and emotional workings and reactions. At the bottom of the inquietude they experience their body as an incomplete source of foundation and of harmony between organic and spiritual values, and more as an insufficient ground for establishing one's identity and place in the world. This is a global *bad mood* related to facticity (the matter-of-factness) as such, primarily directed to one's body. The body as such elicits feelings of disgust, shame, and anxiety, but the meaning of this nebula of feelings must be understood at a more general level. It is the concern for being formless and inconstant in an *existential* sense, that is, featureless, characterless, chaotic, indeterminate as well as discontinuous, unsteady, inconstant, wavering in a temporal sense.

In this chapter we emphasize this fleeting character of emotional life in persons with FED. An interesting perspective is one that sees anorexia, and FED in general, as *passions* (Charland et al., 2013). Passions are long-standing tendencies that represent a rupture in the fleeting and transitory character of emotional life. They represent an abnormal break in the otherwise ceaseless ebb and flow of feeling, which is the more normal state of the events and processes that underlie our emotional life. A passion is a persistent, pervasive, and ego-synthonic emotion that provides a stable normative structure through which a substantial proportion of relations with the environment are evaluated, processed, and responded to. Passions offer fixed points of orientation that endure over time and are incorporated into one's identity (Charland et al., 2013). Once absorbed into one's identity, they move the person to action in often very specifically calculated and defined ways. They suggest interpretations and explanations, and at the same time literally move to action in accordance with fixed goals.

Many passions have a progressive and cumulative course. Sometimes a passion can be so consuming you can't see past it, it is everything you think about, all the time. Passions not only help to direct and organize feelings and emotions, but also cognition. As discussed in Chapter 9, values are attitudes that regulate the felt-meanings of the world and the significant actions of the person, being organized into concepts that do not arise from rational activity but rather within the sphere of feelings. Valuing is a process rooted in the emotional dimension of life. Thus every passion is associated with a fixed intellectual component or idea. The fixed ideas involved in passions are indeed values, or are strongly connected and rooted in values. A person's value system is, first and foremost, a matter of emotional experience, thus of the passions affecting this person. This is also the case with the passion involved in anorexia – *thinness*, which gives to the FED person a steady goal to orientate her life.

Values: Anorexia as a Religion

In some cases, the value in question – thinness – may become obsessive or delusional, although it may not be easy to demonstrate its pathological nature since to do so one may need to formulate a value judgment. In the name of passions, someone may prefer dying for the value of freedom rather than merely surviving in slavery or submission. In anorexia, common-sense priorities are changed: the bodily motive of hunger is outweighed by the motive of shaping up. *Being thin is more important than being healthy*. But one cannot simply take this subversion of common-sense values as a sign of pathology. Debate in recent decades about the boundary between normal and pathological has turned largely on whether and if so in what way it can be defined in value-free terms. Certainly, in the case of anorexic persons, deeming their behavior as pathological implies valuing shaping up a lesser value than survival.

This choice is considered pathological, as well as senseless and incomprehensible, if it is not seen from the angle of a less evident passion in the life of the anorexic person: the passion for having an identity and the need to achieve an identity in an unusual way. From this angle, what is pathological in the life-world of the person affected by anorexia is not her behavior (starvation) or her value (thinness), rather the psychopathological core from which they both arise: an abnormal experience of their own bodily and emotional life.

As we have discussed throughout this chapter, the psychopathological core of the life-world of persons with FED is not feeling oneself coenesthetically, and in particular feeling extraneous from one's body and emotions. This entails a fleeting feeling of selfhood and an evanescent sense of identity. This vulnerable awareness of oneself is disturbing and generates the need to appraise oneself in alternative ways. One of the coping strategies or alternative means of self-recognition in persons with FED is feeling their body through the gaze of others. Obviously, this coping strategy is not voluntarily adopted. A second way to regain a sense of oneself is identifying oneself through one's passion for thinness since passions represent a rupture in the fleeting character of emotional and bodily life. The ossification of this passion and of the related value is the expression of the need to compensate the disturbing, shameful, and anxiogenic fleeting sense of selfhood and identity (Figure 16.1).

If we want to understand what it is like to live with anorexia and bulimia it's a mistake to see ProAna's "philosophy" as merely imperfect cognition or as a kind of irrational or delusional belief about one's body or nutrition. ProAna is a *religion*. Like any religion it lies beyond the rationality/irrationality divide. It is about the worth of life and the way to make one's life meaningful. ProAna is experienced as a faith by its believers. Also it has the same structure of all religions having its own goals, values, creed, rules, and practices. Its goal is authenticity and achieving a place in the world, and more generally the Good Life. The world, one's identity, and place in the world are chaos without Ana. Ana is the savior, a goddess to worship in order to be saved from anarchy and confusion. Food has a moral value: it is a sin and a temptation. Fatness has a moral value too as indicative of laziness, lack of self-care and

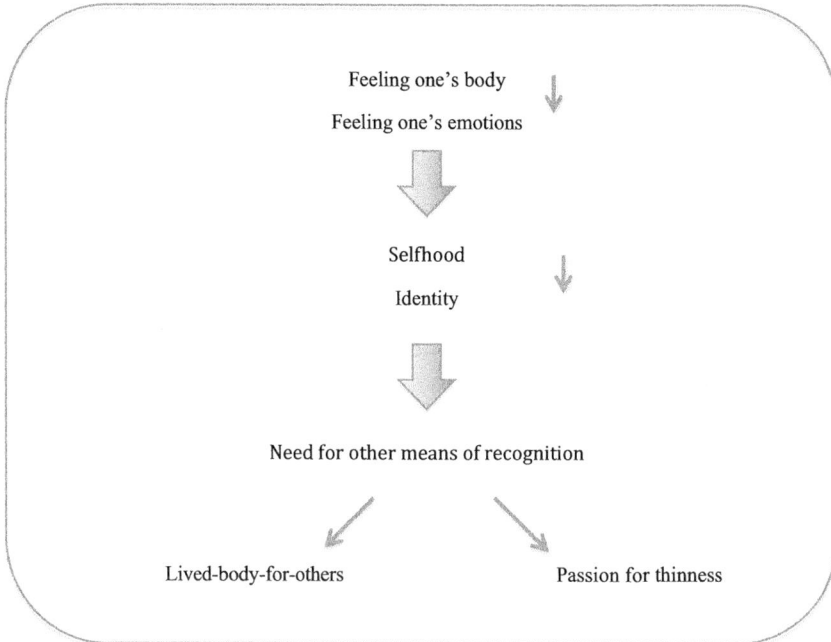

Figure 16.1 Self-recognition in persons with feeding and eating disorders

self-control. Thinness is more valuable than anything else including health. Strict rules are needed not to do wrong and to be led astray. Starvation is the unique salvation practice.

Ana's Creed:

I believe in control, the only force mighty enough to bring order in the chaos that is my world.

I believe that I am the most vile, worthless and useless person ever to have existed on this planet, and that I am totally unworthy of anyone's time and attention.

I believe in oughts, musts and shoulds, as unbreakable laws to determine my daily behavior.

I believe in perfection and strive to attain it.

I believe in salvation through starvation.

I believe in calorie counters as the inspired word of god, and memorize them accordingly.

I believe in bathroom scales as an indicator of my daily successes and failures.

I believe in hell, cause sometimes I think I live in it.

I believe in a wholly black and white world, the losing of weight, recrimination for sins, the alonegation of the body and a life ever fasting.

(*Source*: theproanalifestyleforever)

Ana's Rules:

1. *If you aren't thin you aren't attractive.*
2. *Being thin is more important than being healthy.*
3. *You must buy clothes, style your hair, take laxatives, starve yourself, do anything to make yourself look thinner.*
4. *Thou shall not eat without feeling guilty.*

5. *Thou shall not eat fattening food without punishing oneself afterwards.*
6. *Thou shall count calories and restrict intake accordingly.*
7. *What the scale says is the most important thing.*
8. *Losing weight is good/gaining weight is bad.*
9. *You can never be too thin.*
10. *Being thin and not eating are signs of true will power and success.*
11. *Ana is a lifestyle not a diet*

(*Source*: theproanalifestyleforever.wordpress.com)

ProAna websites and blogs are very good sources for learning what it is like living with anorexia and bulimia. The real issue is understanding the reasons for valuing thinness as absolute goodness. There is an explicit and a covert value in the life-world of persons with FED. The explicit value, as is clear, is thinness. The covert value is the need for identity. Identity has become a task for them due to their alienation from their body and emotion and the lack of a solid and permanent ground to establish it. The transgressive body narratives that can be found in ProAna websites only catch the value of thinness or, as they write, *thinspiration*, not the abnormal lack of identity they stem from.

> Hi sexy skinny Ana's,
> So recently I've been getting a lot of emails about losing weight fast ... Ana is a commitment, it's a disciplined lifestyle and all though we all want to get skinny super fast, it's not the way the world works.
> I'm a firm believer in the idea that we can't choose our path, it chooses us. Ana isn't a diet that you can do a week before your cousins wedding and suddenly magically fit into your bridesmaids dress. It's a commitment. It's a relationship.
> Ana isn't something you can turn on or off. That's why I'm not trying to promote the lifestyle. I'm just helping other fucked up girls like me who are stuck with Ana for the long haul. Whether we like it or not.
> Just thought I would clear this up. You can't find Ana, she finds you.
>
> Stay strong,
> xoxo L
> (*Source*: theproanalifestyleforever.wordpress.com)

ProAna's do not neglect the fact that the value of thinness is related to the need for identity. Yet they seem to miss the connection with estrangement from one's own body and abnormal bodily experiences – the essential psychopathological core of FED. Thus they normalize the value of thinness, defending it as a free choice rather than as a necessity deriving from their alienation from their own lived body. To FED persons, thinness is the achievement of self-control, a move towards success, perfection, and authenticity, that is, the realization of their true identity. The abnormal character of anorexic behavior only comes to light when the values of thinness and self-control are seen as responses to abnormalities of the lived body.

Conclusion

To sum up: in the value system of FED persons being fat (or, in some cases, unfit) has a moral value, not only an aesthetic one. A fat person is a horrible person in the ethical sense of the term. Being fat is perceived as being highly undesirable and having implications for self-worth. Fatness is seen as indicative of laziness, lack of self-care, or lack of self-control,

Table 16.1 The life-world of persons with feeding and eating disorders

Existential	Experiences
Time	Perception of time interconnected with control/loss phases
Body	Wobbling liquid – source of disgust and shame Lived body for others Feeling extraneous from one's bodily self
Other	The mirror through which one can apprehend one's self
Self	Identity as a task Aesthetic or *pornographic* conceptualization of the Self based on seeing and being seen and on the approval of others
Emotions	Shame Disgust Anxiety
Values	Thinness and self-construction Starvation as self-control

and therefore contemptible and disgusting, and likely to lead to unpopularity with peers (Tan et al., 2006a). A fat person is unlovable and a failure. Fat is an indictment of one's entire personality to be avoided at all costs (Tan et al., 2006b). Being thin is more valuable than being healthy or alive. A major shift in values is that the importance of shaping up takes precedence over all or many other aspects of their lives, including health, family, friendships, work, and academic achievement. Starvation is seen as a salvation practice since it can help regain a sense of self-worth and authenticity (Hope et al., 2011).

It's completely useless and inane to oppose these values with common-sense values. There is no way to convince persons with FED that their values are wrong, simply because values may be right or wrong according to the life-world in which they are set. What can be done is helping FED persons to make sense of their passion for thinness and starvation by showing them the core psychopathological anomaly from which it stems – namely, their difficulties in feeling their own body in the first-person perspective and to have a stable and continuous sense of themselves as embodied agents.

The basic concern of FED persons is feeling shapeless in a concrete and metaphorical sense. The value-based therapeutic interview can be a means to accompany them to understand that their set of values and practices are consequences, coping strategies with respect to their lack of the coenesthetic apprehension of their own body as the more primitive and basic form of self-awareness. They will be in a better position to decide whether to continue fighting against a shadow (fatness or physical shapelessness) or to find other, and perhaps more effective, ways to achieve self-recognition and recover a sense of self-identity, that is, to change their concern for being a shapeless body into the care for giving form to their existence.

Table 16.1 summarizes the life-world of persons with feeding and eating disorders.

References

Agamben, G. (2008). *Signatura Rerum: Sul Metodo*. Turin: Bollati Boringhieri.

Akiskal, H. S. (1994). The temperamental borders of affective disorders. *Acta Psychiatica Scandinavica* 379: 32–37.

(1996). The temperamental foundations of mood disorders. In C. Mundt, M. J. Goldstein, K. Hahlweg, and P. Fiedler (eds.), *Interpersonal Factors in the Origin and Course of Affective Disorders*. London: Gaskell, pp. 3–30.

Ambrosini, A., Stanghellini, G., and Langer, A. I. (2010). Typus melancholicus from Tellenbach up to the present day: a review about the premorbid personality vulnerable to melancholia. *Actas Españolas de Psiquiatría* 39: 302–311.

Ambrosini, A., Stanghellini, G., and Raballo, A. (2014). Temperament, personality and the vulnerability to mood disorders: the case of the melancholic type of personality. *Journal of Psychopathology* 20: 393–403.

American Psychiatric Association (2013). *Diagnostic and Statistical Manual of Mental Disorders, Fifth Edition (DSM-5)*. Arlington, VA: American Psychiatric Association.

Ammaniti, M. and Gallese, V. (2014). *The Birth of Intersubjectivity: Psychodynamics, Neurobiology, and the Self*. New York and London: W. W. Norton.

Arbib, M. A. (2007). Other faces in the mirror: a perspective on schizophrenia. *World Psychiatry* 6: 75–78.

Arieti, S. (1959). Manic-depressive psychosis. In S. Arieti (ed.), *American Handbook of Psychiatry*. New York: Basic Books, vol. I, pp. 419–454.

Atwood, G. E. and Stolorow, R. D. (1984). *Structures of Subjectivity: Explorations in Psychoanalytic Phenomenology*. Hillsdale, NJ: Analytic Press.

Ballerini, A. and Stanghellini, G. (1989). Phenomenological questions about obsessions and delusions. *Psychopathology* 22: 315–319.

Ballerini, M. (2016). Autism in schizophrenia: a phenomenological study. In G. Stanghellini and M. Aragona (eds.), *An Experiential Approach to Psychopathology*. New York: Springer, pp. 281–300.

Barthes, R. (2001). *A Lover's Discourse: Fragments*. London: Penguin.

Bayer, R. and Spitzer, R. S. (1985). Neurosis, psychodynamics, and DSM-III: history of the controversy. *Archives of General Psychiatry* 42: 187–196.

Bell, J. (2010). *Redefining Disease: The Harveian Oration*. London: Royal College of Physicians.

Berrios, G. E. (1988). Melancholia and depression during the 19th century: a conceptual history. *British Journal of Psychiatry* 153: 298–304.

(1996). *The History of Mental Symptoms: Descriptive Psychopathology since the Nineteenth Century*. Cambridge University Press.

Berthold-Bond, D. (1995). *Hegel's Theory of Madness*. State University of New York Press.

Berze, J. and Gruhle, H. W. (1929). *Psychologie der Schizophrenie*. Berlin: Springer.

Binswanger, L. (1928/1963). *Being in the World: Selected Papers of Ludwig Binswanger*. New York: Basic Books.

(1960). *Melancholie und manie: Phänomenologische studien*. Pfullingen: Günther Neske.

Blackburn, S. (1998). *Ruling Passions*. Oxford University Press.

Blankenburg, W. (1969). Ansaetze zu einer Psychopathologie des "common sense." *Confinia Psychiatrica* 12: 144–163.

(1971). *Der Verlust der natürlichen Selbstverständlichkeit: Ein Beitrag zur Psychopathologie symptomarmer*

Schizophrenien. Stuttgart: Ferdinand Enke Verlag.

Bollas, C. (2003). *Being a Character: Psychoanalysis and Self-Experience*. London: Routledge.

Brakel, L. A. W. (2009). *Philosophy, Psychoanalysis, and the A-rational Mind*. Oxford University Press.

Bradshaw, J. (1994). *Creating Love: The Next Great Stage of Growth*. New York: Bantam.

Buber, M. (1958). *I and Thou*. New York: Scribner.

Bürgy, M. (2007). Prolegomena zu einer Psychopathologie der Verzweiflung. *Der Nervenarzt* 78: 521–529.

Buytendijk, F. J. (1988). The first smile of the child. *Phenomenology and Pedagogy* 6: 15–24.

Callieri, B. (2001). *Quando vince l'ombra: problemi di psicopatologia clinica*. Rome: Edizioni Universitarie Romane.

Callieri, B., Maldonato, M., and Di Petta, G. (1999). *Lineamenti di psicopatologia fenomenologica*. Naples: Alfredo Guida Editore.

Calvi, L. (2005). *Il Tempo dell'altro Significato*. Milan: Mimesis.

Cassano, G. B., Dell'Osso, L., Frank, E., Miniati, M., Fagiolini, A., Shear, K., Pini, S., and Maser, J. (1999). The bipolar spectrum: a clinical reality in search of diagnostic criteria and an assessment methodology. *Journal of Affective Disorders* 54: 319–328.

Castellini, G., Franzago, M., Bagnoli, S., Lelli L., Balsamo, M., Mancini, M. *et al.* (2017). Fat mass and obesity-associated gene (FTO) is associated to eating disorders susceptibility and moderates the expression of psychopathological traits. *PloS ONE* 12: e0173560.

Castellini, G., Stanghellini, G., Godini, L., Lucchese, M., Trisolini, F., and Ricca, V. (2015). Abnormal bodily experiences mediate the relationship between impulsivity and binge eating in overweight subjects seeking bariatric surgery. *Psychotherapy and Psychosomatics* 84: 124–126.

Castellini, G., Trisolini, F., and Ricca, V. (2014). Psychopathology of eating disorders. *Journal of Psychopathology* 20: 461–470.

Charland, L. C., Hope, T., Stewart, A., and Tan, J. (2013). The hypothesis that anorexia nervosa is a passion: clarifications and elaborations. *Philosophy, Psychiatry, & Psychology* 20: 375–379.

Clark, A. (1997). *Being There: Putting Brain, Body, and World Together Again*. Cambridge, MA: MIT Press.

Cloninger, C. R. (1994). Temperament and personality. *Current Opinion in Neurobiology* 4: 266–273.

Conrad, K. (1966). *Die beginnende Schizophrenie: versuch einer Gestaltanalyse des Wahns*. Stuttgart: Thieme.

Correale, A. (2007). *Area traumatica e campo istituzionale*, 2nd edition. Rome: Borla Edizioni.

Costa, C., Carmenates, S., Madeira, L., and Stanghellini, G. (2014). Phenomenology of atmospheres: the felt meanings of clinical encounters. *Journal of Psychopathology* 20: 351–357.

Damasio, A. R. (2004). Emotions and feelings: a neurobiological perspective. In A. S. R. Manstead, N. Frijda, and A. Fischer (eds.), *Feelings and Emotions: The Amsterdam Symposium*. Cambridge University Press, pp. 49–57.

De Martino, E. (1997). *Il mondo magico: prolegomeni a una storia del magismo*. Turin: Bollati Boringhieri.

(2002). Promesse e minacce dell'etnologia. In E. De Martino (ed.), *Furore Simbolo Valore*. Milan: Feltrinelli, pp. 84–118.

De Sousa, R. (2011). *Emotional Truth*. Oxford University Press.

Dillon, M. C. (1997). *Merleau-Ponty's Ontology*. Evanston, IL: Northwestern University Press.

Dörr-Zegers, O. (1993). El cambio de la corporalidad y su importancia para la determinación de un síndrome depresivo fundamental o nuclear. *Revista de psiquiatría de la Facultad de Medicina de Barcelona* 20: 202–212.

(1995). *Psiquiatría Antropológica: contribuciones a una Psiquiatría de orientación fenomenológica-antropológica*. Santiago de Chile: Editorial Universitaria.

Dörr-Zegers, O. and Stanghellini, G. (2015). Phenomenology of corporeality: a paradigmatic case study in schizophrenia. *Actas Españolas de Psiquiatría* 43: 1–7.

Dörr-Zegers, O. and Tellenbach, H. (1980). Differential phenomenology of depressive states. *Der Nervenarzt* 51: 113–118.

Eddy, K. T., Dorer, D. J., Franko, D. L., Tahilani, K., Thompson-Brenner, H., and Herzog, D. B. (2008). Diagnostic crossover in anorexia nervosa and bulimia nervosa: implications for DSM-V. *American Journal of Psychiatry* 165: 245–250.

Endicott, J. and Spitzer, R. (1978). A diagnostic interview schedule for affective disorders and schizophrenia. *Archives of General Psychiatry* 35: 837–844.

Ey, H. (1959). Los delirios. *Revista de Psiquiatría del Uruguay* 140: 3–42.

Ey, H., Bernard, P., and Brisset, C. (1960). *Manuel de psychiatrie*. Paris: Masson.

Fairburn, C. G. and Cooper, Z. (2007). Thinking afresh about the classification of eating disorders. *International Journal of Eating Disorders* 40: S107–S110.

Fairburn, C. G., Cooper, Z., and Shafran, R. (2003). Cognitive behaviour therapy for eating disorders: a "transdiagnostic" theory and treatment. *Behaviour Research and Therapy* 41: 509–528.

Fenichel, O. (1945). *Psychoanalytic Theory of the Neuroses*. New York: W. W. Norton.

Fernandez, A. V. (2016). Language, prejudice and the aims of hermeneutic phenomenology. In G. Stanghellini, L. A. Sass, E. Pienkos, and G. Castellini (eds.), *Language and Psychopathology*. Special issue of *Journal of Psychopathology* 22: 21–29.

Finn, S. E. and Tonsanger, M. E. (1997). Information gathering and therapeutic models of assessment: complementary paradigms. *Psychological Assessment* 9: 374–385.

Fiorillo, A., Sampogna, G., Del Vecchio, V., Luciano, M., Ambrosini, A., and Stanghellini, G. (2016). Education in psychopathology in Europe: results from a survey in 32 countries. *Academic Psychiatry* 40: 242–248.

Fonagy, P. and Target, M. (1997). Attachment and reflective function: their role in self-organization. *Development and Psychopathology* 9: 679–700.

Foucault, M. (2003). *Le pouvoir psychiatrique*. Paris: Seuil.

Freeman, L. and Elpidorou, A. (2015). Affectivity in Heidegger II: temporality, boredom, and beyond. *Philosophy Compass* 10: 672–684.

Freud, S. (1905). *Three Essays on the Theory of Sexuality*. Standard Edition of the Complete Psychological Works of Sigmund Freud, vol. 7. London: Hogarth Press.

(1926). *Inhibition, Symptoms and Anxiety*. Standard Edition of the Complete Psychological Works of Sigmund Freud, vol. 20. London: Hogarth Press.

Fuchs, T. (2001). Melancholia as a desynchronization: towards a psychopathology of interpersonal time. *Psychopathology* 34: 179–186.

(2002). The phenomenology of shame, guilt and the body in body dysmorphic disorder and depression. *Journal of Phenomenological Psychology* 33: 223–243.

(2005). The phenomenology of body, space and time in depression. *Comprendre* 15: 108–121.

(2007). Fragmented selves: temporality and identity in borderline personality. *Psychopathology* 40: 379–387.

(2010). Phenomenology and psychopathology. In D. Schmicking and S. Gallagher (eds.), *Handbook of Phenomenology and Cognitive Science*. Dordrecht: Springer, pp. 547–573.

(2013a). Temporality and psychopathology. *Phenomenology and the Cognitive Sciences* 12: 75–104.

(2013b). The self in schizophrenia: Jaspers, Schneider, and beyond. In G. Stanghellini and T. Fuchs (eds.), *One Century of Karl Jaspers' General Psychopathology*. Oxford University Press, pp. 245–257.

(2013c). Existential vulnerability: towards a psychopathology of limit situation. *Psychopathology* 46: 301–308.

(2014). Psychopathology of depression and mania: symptoms, phenomena and syndromes. *Journal of Psychopathology* 20: 404–413.

Fulford, K. W. M. (1999). *Moral Theory and Medical Practice*. Cambridge University Press.

Fulford, K. W. M. and Stanghellini, G. (forthcoming). Values and values-based practice. In G. Stanghellini *et al.* (eds.), *The Oxford Handbook of Phenomenological Psychopathology*. Oxford University Press.

Gabbani, C. and Stanghellini, G. (2008). What kind of objectivity do we need for psychiatry? A commentary to Oulis's ontological assumptions in psychiatric taxonomy. *Psychopathology* 41: 203–204.

Gadamer, H. G. (2004). *Truth and Method*, trans. J. Weinsheimer and D. G. Marshall, 2nd revised edition. New York: Continuum.

Gallagher, S. (2005). *How the Body Shapes the Mind*. Oxford University Press.

Gallagher, S. and Zahavi, D. (2012). *The Phenomenological Mind*, 2nd edition. London and New York: Routledge.

Gallese, V. and Goldman, A. (1998). Mirror neurons and the simulation theory of mind-reading. *Trends in Cognitive Sciences* 2: 493–501.

Glass, G. (2003). Anxiety: animal reactions and the embodiment of meaning. In K. W. M. Fulford, K. Morris, J. Z. Sadler, and G. Stanghellini (eds.), *Nature and Narrative: An Introduction to the New Philosophy of Psychiatry*. Oxford University Press, pp. 231–249.

Goldie, P. (2000). *Emotions: A Philosophical Exploration*. Oxford University Press.

Gray, J. (2010). *Gray's Anatomy*. London: Penguin.

Grinberg, L. (1964). Two kinds of guilt: their relations with normal and pathological aspects of mourning. *International Journal of Psychoanalysis* 45: 366–371.

Grøn, A. (2004). Self and identity. In D. Zahavi, T. Grünbaum, and J. Parnas (eds.), *Structure and Development of Self-Consciousness: Interdisciplinary Perspectives*. Philadelphia, PA: John Benjamins, pp. 123–156.

Gross, G., Huber, G., Klosterkötter, J., and Linz, M. (1987). *BSABS Bonner Skala für die Beurteilung von Basissymptomen*. Berlin: Springer Verlag.

Gunderson, J. G. and Phillips, K. A. (1991). A current view of the interface between borderline personality disorder and depression. *American Journal of Psychiatry* 148: 967–975.

Hales, R. E. and Yudofsky, S. C. (1999). *Essentials of Clinical Psychiatry*. Washington, DC: American Psychiatric Press.

Hales, R. E., Yudofsky, S. C., and Tallbot, J. A. (1999). *Textbook of Psychiatry*, 3rd edition. Washington, DC: American Psychiatric Press.

Heidegger, M. (1927/1962). *Being and Time*. Oxford: Blackwell.

(2001). *The Fundamental Concepts of Metaphysics: World, Finitude, Solitude*. Bloomington, IN: Indiana University Press.

Henriksen, M. G. and Parnas, J. (2012). Clinical manifestations of self-disorders and the Gestalt of schizophrenia. *Schizophrenia Bulletin* 38: 657–660.

Henry, M. (1973). *The Essence of Manifestation*. The Hague: Martinus Nijhoff.

Herran, A., Sierra-Biddle, D., de Santiago, A., Artal, J., Diez-Manrique, J. F., and Vazquez-Barquero, J. L. (2001). Diagnostic accuracy in the first five minutes of a psychiatric interview. *Psychotherapy and Psychosomatics* 70: 141–144.

Honneth, A. (2008). Reconnaissance et reproduction sociale. In J. P. Payet and A. Battegay (eds.), *La reconnaissance à l'épreuve. Explorations socio-anthropologiques*. Villeneuve d'Ascq: Presses Universitaires du Septentrion, pp. 45–58.

Hope, T., Tan, J., Stewart, A., and Fitzpatrick, R. (2011). Anorexia nervosa and the language of authenticity. *Hastings Center Report* 41: 19–29.

Hopkinson, K., Cox, A., and Rutter, M. (1981). Psychiatric interviewing techniques III. Naturalistic study: eliciting feelings. *British Journal of Psychiatry* 138: 406–415.

Huber, G. (1957). Die coenaesthetische schizophrenie. *Fortschritte der Neurologie Psychiatrie* 25: 491–520.

(1983). Das Konzept substratnaher Basissymptome und seine Bedeutung für Theorie und Therapie schizophrener Erkrankungen. *Der Nervenarzt* 54: 23–32.

(1995). Prodrome der Schizophrenie. *Fortschritte der Neurologie Psychiatrie* 63: 131–138.

Huber, G., Gross, G., and Schüttler, R. (1979). *Schizophrenie: Eine Verlaufs-und sozialpsychiatrische Langzeituntersuchungen.* Berlin: Springer.

Husserl, E. (1912–1915). *Ideen zu einer reinen Phaenomenologie und phaenomenologische Philosophie. II. Phaenomenologische Untersuchungen zur Konstitution.* The Hague: Martinus Nijhoff.

(1936/1970). *The Crisis of European Sciences and Transcendental Phenomenology: An Introduction to Phenomenological Philosophy.* Evanston, IL: Northwestern University Press.

(1950). *Cartesianische meditationen und Pariser Vorträge.* Husserliana 1. The Hague: Martinus Nijhoff.

(1977). Seeing essences as genuine method for grasping the a priori. In E. Husserl, *Phenomenological Psychology.* The Hague: Martinus Nijhff, pp. 53–64.

(1988). *Vorlesungen über Ethik und Wertlehre (1908–1914).* Husserliana 28. Dordrecht: Kluwer.

(1991). *On the Phenomenology of the Consciousness of Internal Time.* Dordrecht: Kluwer.

(2002). *Zur Phänomenologischen Reduktionen. Texte aus dem Nachlass (1926–1935),* ed. Sebastian Luft. Husserliana 34. Dordrecht: Kluwer.

Hutto, D. D. (2007). The narrative practice hypothesis: origins and application of folk psychology. In D. D. Hutto (ed.), *Narrative and Understanding Persons.* Cambridge University Press, pp. 43–88.

(2013). Interpersonal relating. In K. W. M. Fulford, M. Davies, R. G. T. Gipps, G.

Graham, J. Z. Sadler, G. Stanghellini, and T. Thornton (eds.), *The Oxford Handbook of Philosophy and Psychiatry.* Oxford University Press, pp. 249–257.

Ingram, D. H. (1979). Time and timekeeping in psychoanalysis and psychotherapy. *American Journal of Psychoanalysis* 39: 319–328.

Jaspers, K. (1913/1997). *General Psychopathology,* trans. J. Hoenig and M. W. Hamilton. Baltimore, MD: Johns Hopkins University Press.

(1925). *Psychologie der Weltanschauungen.* Berlin: Springer.

Jay, M. (1994). *Downcast Eyes: The Denigration of Vision in Twentieth-Century French Thought.* Berkeley and Los Angeles, CA: University of California Press.

Johnson, S. C. (2000). The recognition of mentalistic agents in infancy. *Trends in Cognitive Sciences* 4: 22–28.

Jouvent, R. and Widlocher, D. (1994). Les théories psychologiques, la vulnérabilité et la dépression. *Encephale* 4: 639–643.

Kane, S. (2001). *4.48 Psychosis.* In S. Kane, *Complete Plays.* London: Methuen, pp. 203–246.

Kaplan, H. I. and Sadock, B. J. (2005). *Comprehensive Textbook of Psychiatry,* 7th edition. Baltimore, MD: Lippincott Williams & Wilkins.

Kendler, K. S. (2008). Introduction: why does psychiatry need philosophy? In K. S. Kendler and J. Parnas (eds.), *Philosophical Issues in Psychiatry: Explanation, Phenomenology, and Nosology.* Baltimore, MD: Johns Hopkins University Press, pp. 1–16.

Kendler, K. S. and Parnas. J. (eds.) (2008). *Philosophical Issues in Psychiatry: Explanation, Phenomenology, and Nosology.* Baltimore, MD: Johns Hopkins University Press.

Kendler, K. S. and Parnas (2012). *Philosophical Issues in Psychiatry II: Nosology.* Oxford University Press.

Kernberg, O. F. (1984). The couch at sea: psychoanalytic studies of group and organizational leadership. *International Journal of Group Psychotherapy* 34: 5–23.

Kimura, B. (1992). *Écrits de psychopathologie phénoménologique*, trans. J. Bouderlique. Paris: Presses Universitaires de France.

(2000). *L'Entre. Une approche phénoménologique de la schizophrénie*, trans. C. Vincent. Grenoble: Éditions Jérôme Millon.

Kirk, S. A. and Kutchins, H. (1992). *The Selling of the DSM: The Rhetoric of Science in Psychiatry*. New York: Aldine de Gruyter.

Klosterkötter, J. (1988). *Basissymptome und Endphaenomene der Schizophrenie*. Berlin: Springer.

(1992). The meaning of basic symptoms for the genesis of the schizophrenic nuclear syndrome. *Psychiatry and Clinical Neurosciences* 46: 609–630.

Kraus, A. (1977). *Sozialverhalten und Psychose Manisch-Depressiver*. Stuttgart: Enke.

(1982). Identity and psychosis of the manic-depressive. In A. J. A. De Koning and F. A. Jenner (eds.), *Phenomenology and Psychiatry*. London: Academic Press, pp. 201–216.

(1987). Dynamique du rôle des maniaques-dépressifs et conséquences thérapeutiques. *Psychologie Médicale* 19: 401–405.

(1991). Modes d'existence des hystériques et des mélancoliques. In P. Fédida and J. Schotte (eds.), *Psychiatrie et existence*. Grenoble: Millon, pp. 263–280.

(1994). Le motif du mensonge et la dépersonnalisation dans la mélancholie. *Evolution psychiatrique* 59: 6349–6357.

(1995). Psychotherapy based on identity problems of depressives. *American Journal of Psychotherapy* 49: 197–212.

(1996). Role performance, identity structure and psychosis in melancholic and manic-depressive patients. In C. H. Mundt (ed.), *Interpersonal Factors in the Origin and Course of Affective Disorders*. London: Gaskell, pp. 31–47.

(2003). How can the phenomenological-anthropological approach contribute to diagnosis and classification in psychiatry? In K. W. M. Fulford, K. Morris, J. Z. Sadler, and G. Stanghellini (eds.), *Nature and Narrative: An Introduction to the New Philosophy of Psychiatry*. Oxford University Press, pp. 199–216.

Kretschmer, E. (1919). *Der sensitive Beziehungswahn. Ein Beitrag zur Paranoidefrage und zur psychiatrischen Charakterlehre*. Berlin: Springer.

(1921/1961). *Korperbau und Charakter*. Berlin: Springer.

Kupke, C. (2005). Lived time and to live time: a critical comment on a paper by Martin Wyllie. *Philosophy, Psychiatry, & Psychology* 12: 199–203.

Lacan, J. (2005). *Le Seminaire Livre XXIII. Le Synthome (1975–76)*. Paris: Seuil.

Laing, R. D. (2010). *The Divided Self: An Existential Study in Sanity and Madness*. London: Penguin.

Lakoff, G. and Johnson, M. (2008). *Metaphors We Live By*. University of Chicago Press.

Lange, J. (1926). Ueber Melancholie. *Zeitschrift für die gesammte Neurologie und Psichiatrie* 101: 293–301.

Lanteri-Laura, G. (1993). Introduction à l'oeuvre psychopathologique d'Eugène Minkowski (Postface). In E. Minkowski, *Structure des depressions*. Paris: Nouvel Object.

Lazarsfeld, P. F. (1935). The art of asking WHY in marketing research: three principles underlying the formulation of questionnaires. *National Marketing Review* 1: 26–38.

LeDoux, J. E. (2000). Cognitive-emotional interactions: listen to the brain. In R. D. Lane and L. Nadel (eds.), *Cognitive Neuroscience of Emotion*. Oxford University Press, pp. 129–155.

Leoni, F. (2008). *Habeas Corpus: Sei Genealogie del Corpo Occidentale*. Milan: Bruno Mondadori.

Leopardi, G. (1992). *Zibaldone: A Selection*. New York: Peter Lang.

(2002). *Thoughts: And, The Broom [or The Flower of the Desert]*. London: Hesperus Press.

Levin, D. M. (1993). *Modernity and the Hegemony of Vision*. Berkeley and Los Angeles, CA: University of California Press.

Lieberman, P. B. (1989). Objective methods and subjective experiences. *Schizophrenia Bulletin* 15: 267–275.

López-Ibor, J. J. Jr. (1974). *El cuerpo y la corporalidad*. Madrid: Gredos.

Mackinnon, R. A. and Michels, R. (1971). *The Psychiatric Interview in Clinical Practice*. Philadelphia, PA: Saunders.

Mayer-Gross, W., Slater, E., and Roth, M. (1954). *Clinical Psychiatry*. London: Cassell.

McDougall, J. (1996). *Theatres of the Body*. London: Free Association Books.

McGuffin, P. and Farmer, A. (2001). Polydiagnostic approaches to measuring and classifying psychopathology. *American Journal of Medical Genetics* 105: 39–41.

Meares, R. (2000). *Intimacy and Alienation: Memory, Trauma and Personal Being*. London: Routledge.

Merleau-Ponty, M. (1945/1962). *The Phenomenology of Perception*. London: Routledge & Kegan Paul.

Miller, J. A. (1998). *Le symptôme charlatan*. Paris: Seuil.

Milos, G., Spindler, A., Schnyder, U., and Fairburn, C. G. (2005). Instability of eating disorder diagnoses: prospective study. *British Journal of Psychiatry* 187: 573–578.

Minkowski, E. (1927). *La Schizophrénie: Psychopathologie des schizoïdes et des Schizophrènes*. Paris: Payot.

(1930/1993). Etude sur la structure des états de dépression: les depréssions ambivalentes. In E. Minkowski, *Structure des dépressions*. Paris: Nouvel Object.

(1933/1970). *Lived Time*. Evanston, IL: Northwestern University Press.

Mishler, E. G. (1986). *Research Interviewing: Context and Narrative*. Cambridge, MA: Harvard University Press.

Mond, J. M., Latner, J. D., Hay, P. H., Owen, C., and Rodgers, B. (2010). Objective and subjective bulimic episodes in the classification of bulimic-type eating disorders: another nail in the coffin of a problematic distinction. *Behaviour Research and Therapy* 48: 661–669.

Monti, M. R. and Stanghellini, G. (1996). Psychopathology: an edgeless razor? *Comprehensive Psychiatry* 37: 196–204.

Mooij, A. (2012). *Psychiatry as a Human Science: Phenomenological, Hermeneutic and Lacanian Perspectives*. Amsterdam: Rodopi.

Mullen, P. E. and Fergusson, D. M. (1999). *Childhood Sexual Abuse: An Evidence-Based Perspective*. Thousand Oaks, CA: Sage Publications.

Mundt, C., Golstein, M. J., Halweg, K., and Fiedler, P. (1996). *Interpersonal Factors in the Origin and Course of Affective Disorders*. London: Gaskell.

Nordbø, R. H., Espeset, E. M., Gulliksen, K. S., and Holte, A. (2006). The meaning of self-starvation: qualitative study of patients' perception of anorexia nervosa. *International Journal of Eating Disorders* 39: 556–564.

Northoff, G. (2014). *Minding the Brain: A Guide to Philosophy and Neuroscience*. Basingstoke: Palgrave Macmillan.

(2016a). How do resting state changes in depression translate into psychopathological symptoms? From "spatiotemporal correspondence" to "spatiotemporal psychopathology." *Current Opinion in Psychiatry* 29: 18–24.

(2016b). Spatiotemporal psychopathology II. How does a psychopathology of the brain's resting state look like? Spatiotemporal approach and the history of psychopathology. *Journal of Affective Disorders* 190: 867–879.

Northoff, G. and Stanghellini, G. (2016). How to link brain and experience? Spatiotemporal psychopathology of the lived body. *Frontiers in Human Neuroscience* 28: 10–76.

Othmer, E. and Othmer, S. C. (2002). *The Clinical Interview Using DSM-IV, Vol. 1: Fundamentals*. Washington, DC: American Psychiatric Publishing.

Oyebode, F. (2008). *Sim's Symptoms in the Mind: An Introduction to Descriptive Psychopathology*. Edinburgh: Saunders-Elsevier.

Pallasmaa, J. (1999). Hapticity and time. *Architectural Review* 207: 78–84.

Panksepp, J. (2005a). On the embodied neural nature of core emotional affects. *Journal of Consciousness Studies* 12: 158–184.

(2005b). Affective consciousness: core emotional feelings in animals and humans. *Cognition and Consciousness* 14: 30–80.

Paris, J. (1994). *Borderline Personality Disorder: A Multidimensional Approach.* Washington, DC: American Psychiatric Press.

(2000). *Myths of Childhood.* Philadelphia, PA: Brunner/Mazel.

Parnas, J. (2005). Clinical detection of schizophrenia-prone individuals. *British Journal of Psychiatry* 187: S111–S112.

Parnas, J., Jansson, L., Sass, L. A., and Handest, P. (1998). Self-experience in the prodromal phases of schizophrenia: a pilot study of first-admissions. *Neurology, Psychiatry and Brain Research* 6: 97–106.

Parnas, J., Møller, P., Kircher, T., and Zahavi, D. (2005). EASE: examination of anomalous self-experience. *Psychopathology* 38: 236–258.

Parnas, J. and Sass, L. A. (2011). The structure of self-consciousness in schizophrenia. In S. Gallagher (ed.), *The Oxford Handbook of the Self.* Oxford University Press, pp. 521–546.

Pazzagli, A. and Monti, M. (2000). Dysphoria and aloneness in borderline personality disorder. *Psychopathology* 33: 220–226.

PDM Task Force (2006). *Psychodynamic Diagnostic Manual.* Silver Spring, MD: Alliance of Psychoanalytic Organizations.

Perugi, G., Akiskal, H. S., Lattanzi, L., Cecconi, D., Mastrocinque, C., Patronelli, A., Vignoli, S., and Bemi, E. (1998). The high prevalence of "soft" bipolar (II) features in atypical depression. *Comprehensive Psychiatry* 39: 63–71.

Peters, L. and Andrews, G. (1995). The procedural validity of the computerized version of the Composite International Diagnostic Interview. *Psychological Medicine* 25: 1269–1280.

Phillips, J. (2003). Schizophrenia and the narrative self. In T. Kircher and A. David (eds.), *The Self in Neuroscience and Psychiatry.* Cambridge University Press, pp. 319–335.

Phillips, M. L., Senior, C., Fahy, T., and David, A. S. (1998). Disgust: the forgotten emotion in psychiatry. *British Journal of Psychiatry* 172: 373–375.

Phillips, M. L., Young, A. W., Senior, C., ... and David, A. S. (1997). A specific neural substrate for perceiving facial expressions of disgust. *Nature* 389: 495–498.

Pickard, H. (2013). Responsibility without blame: philosophical reflections on clinical practice. In K. W. M. Fulford, M. Davies, R. G. T. Gipps, G. Graham, J. Z. Sadler, G. Stanghellini, and T. Thornton (eds.), *The Oxford Handbook of Philosophy and Psychiatry.* Oxford University Press, pp. 1134–1154.

Pidgeon, N. and Henwood, K. (1996). Grounded theory: practical implementation. In J. T. Richardson (ed.), *Handbook of Qualitative Research Methods for Psychology and the Social Sciences.* Leicester: British Psychological Society, pp. 86–101.

Plutchik, R. (1980). *Emotion: A Psychoevolutionary Synthesis.* New York: Harper & Row.

Pollio, H. R., Henley, T., and Thompson, C. B. (1997). *The Phenomenology of Everyday Life.* Cambridge University Press.

Pollock, D. C., Shanley, D. F., and Byrne, P. N. (1985). Psychiatric interviewing and clinical skills. *Canadian Journal of Psychiatry* 30: 64–68.

Prinz, J. (2005). Are emotions feelings? *Journal of Consciousness Studies* 12: 9–25.

Ratcliffe, M. and Stephan, A. (2014). *Depression, Emotion and the Self: Philosophical and Interdisciplinary Perspectives.* Exeter: Imprint Academic.

Ricca, V., Castellini, G., Mannucci, E., Sauro, C. L., Ravaldi, C., Rotella, C. M., and Faravelli, C. (2010). Comparison of individual and group cognitive behavioral therapy for binge eating disorder: a randomized, three-year follow-up study. *Appetite* 55: 656–665.

Richardson, J. T. (ed.) (1996). *Handbook of Qualitative Research Methods for Psychology and the Social Sciences.* Leicester: British Psychological Society.

Ricoeur, P. (1950). *Philosophie de la volonté, vol. 1: Le Volontaire et l'Involontaire*. Paris: Seuil.

(1960). *The Philosophy of the Will, vol. 2: Fallible Man*. New York: Fordham University Press.

(1981). *Hermeneutics and the Human Sciences*, trans. and ed. J. B. Thompson. Cambridge University Press.

(1992). *Oneself as Another*. University of Chicago Press.

(2004). *Parcours de la Reconnaissance*. Paris: Stock.

Rilke, R. M. (1910/1990). *The Notebooks of Malte Laurids Brigge*. New York: Vintage International.

Rochat, P. (2001). *The Infant's World*. Cambridge, MA: Harvard University Press.

Rorty, R. (1981). *Philosophy and the Mirror of Nature*. Princeton University Press.

Rosch, E. (1975). Cognitive reference point. *Cognitive Psychology* 7: 532–547.

Rosfort, R. and Stanghellini, G. (2009). The person in between moods and affects. *Philosophy, Psychiatry, & Psychology* 16: 251–266.

Rossi Monti, M. and D'Agostino, A. (2014). Borderline personality disorder from a psychopathological-dynamic perspective. *Journal of Psychopathology* 20: 451–460.

Russell, J. A. (2003). Core affect and the psychological construction of emotion. *Psychological Review* 110: 145–172.

Rutter, M. (1987). Temperament, personality, and personality disorder. *British Journal of Psychiatry* 150: 443–458.

Sadler, J. Z. (2005). *Values and Psychiatric Diagnosis*. Oxford University Press.

Sadler, J. Z., Hulgus, Y. F., and Agich, G. J. (1994). On values in recent American psychiatric classification. *Journal of Medical Philosophy* 19: 261–277.

Saghir, M. T. (1971). A comparison of some aspects of structured and unstructured psychiatric interviews. *American Journal of Psychiatry* 128: 180–184.

Sartre, J.-P. (1939). *Esquisse d'une théorie des émotions*. Paris: Hermann.

(1943/1992). *Being and Nothingness*. New York: Washington Square Press.

Sass, L. A. (2001). Self and world in schizophrenia: three classic approaches. *Philosophy, Psychiatry, & Psychology* 8: 251–270.

(2004). Affectivity in schizophrenia: a phenomenological view. *Journal of Consciousness Studies* 11: 127–147.

Sass, L. A. and Parnas, J. (2003). Schizophrenia, consciousness, and the self. *Schizophrenia Bulletin* 29: 427–444.

Sass, L. and Pienkos, E. (2013a). Varieties of self-experience: a comparative phenomenology of melancholia, mania, and schizophrenia, Part I. *Journal of Consciousness Studies* 20: 103–130.

(2013b). Space, time, and atmosphere: a comparative phenomenology of melancholia, mania, and schizophrenia, Part II. *Journal of Consciousness Studies* 20: 131–152.

Sassaroli, S., Gallucci, M., and Ruggiero, G. M. (2008). Low perception of control as a cognitive factor of eating disorders: its independent effects on measures of eating disorders and its interactive effects with perfectionism and self-esteem. *Journal of Behavior Therapy and Experimental Psychiatry* 39: 467–488.

Scheler, M. (1927/1973). *Formalism in Ethics and Non-Formal Ethics of Values*. Evanston, IL: Northwestern University Press.

(1928/2012). *Person and Self-Value: Three Essays*. Dordrecht: Springer.

(1973). Wesen und Formen der Sympathie. In M. Scheler, *Gesammelte Werke*. Band 7. Bern: Francke Verlag.

(2008). *The Constitution of the Human Being: From the Posthumous Works, Volumes 11 and 12*. Milwaukee, WI: Marquette University Press.

Schneider, K. (1920). Die Schichtung des emotionalen Lebens und der Aufbau der Depressionszustände. *Zeitschrift für die gesamte Neurologie und Psychiatrie* 59: 281–286.

(1935). *Pathopsyhologie der Gefühle und Triebe*. Leipzig: Georg Thieme Verlag.

(1950). *Klinische psychopathologie*. Stuttgart: Georg Thieme.

Schulte, W. (1961). Nichttraurigseinkönnen im Kern melancholischen Erlebens. *Nervenarzt* 32: 314–320.

Schutz, A. and Luckmann, T. (1973). *The Structures of the Life-World, Volume I*. Evanston, IL: Northwestern University Press.

(1989). *The Structures of the Life-World, Volume II*. Evanston, IL: Northwestern University Press.

Schwartz, M. A. and Wiggins, O. P. (1987). Typifications: the first step for clinical diagnosis in psychiatry. *Journal of Nervous and Mental Disease* 175: 65–77.

Segrott, J. and Doel, M. (2004). Disturbing geography: obsessive-compulsive disorder as spatial practice. *Social & Cultural Geography* 5: 597–614.

Shea, S. C. (1988). *Psychiatric Interviewing: The Art of Understanding*. Philadelphia, PA: Saunders.

Shea, S. C. and Mezzich, J. E. (1988). Contemporary psychiatric interviewing: new directions for training. *Psychiatry* 51: 385–397.

Sheets-Johnstone, M. (1999a). Emotion and movement: a beginning empirical-phenomenological analysis of their relationship. *Journal of Consciousness Studies* 6: 259–277.

(1999b). *The Primacy of Movement*. Amsterdam: John Benjamins.

Shimoda, M. (1950). On manic-depressive illness [in Japanese]. *Yonago Igakushi* 2: 62.

Siemer, M. (2005). Moods as multiple-object directed and as objectless affective states: an examination of the dispositional theory of moods. *Cognition and Emotion* 19: 815–845

Skarderud, F. (2007a). Eating one's words, part I. "Concretised metaphors" and reflective function in anorexia nervosa: an interview study. *European Eating Disorders Review* 15: 163–174.

(2007b). Eating one's words, part II. The embodied mind and reflective function in anorexia nervosa: theory. *European Eating Disorders Review* 15: 243–252.

Smith, Q. (1986). *The Felt Meanings of the World: A Metaphysics of Feeling*. West Lafayette, IN: Purdue University Press.

Smolik, P. (1999). Validity of nosological classification. *Dialogues in Clinical Neuroscience* 1: 185–190.

Solomon, R. C. (2007). *True To Our Feelings: What Our Emotions Are Really Telling Us*. Oxford University Press.

Spitzer, R. L. (1983). Psychiatric diagnosis: are clinicians still necessary? *Comprehensive Psychiatry* 24: 399–411.

(2001). Values and assumptions in the development of DSM-III-R: an insider's perspective and a belated response to Sadler, Hulgus, and Agich's "On values in recent American psychiatric classification." *Journal of Nervous & Mental Disease* 189: 351–359.

Stanghellini, G. (1997). *Antropologia della vulnerabilità*. Milan: Feltrinelli.

(2000a). The doublets of anger. *Psychopathology* 33: 155–158.

(2000b). Vulnerability to schizophrenia and lack of common sense. *Schizophrenia Bulletin* 26: 775–787.

(2000c). Phenomenology of the social self of the schizotype and the melancholic type. In D. Zahavi (ed.), *Exploring the Self: Philosophical and Psychopathological Perspectives on Self-Experience*. Amsterdam: John Benjamins, pp. 279–294.

(2001). Psychopathology of common sense. *Philosophy, Psychiatry, & Psychology* 8: 201–218.

(2004). The puzzle of the psychiatric interview. *Journal of Phenomenological Psychology* 35: 173–195.

(2005). For an anthropology of eating disorders: a pornographic vision of the self. *Eating and Weight Disorders* 10: 21–27.

(2007). The grammar of the psychiatric interview. *Psychopathology* 40: 69–74.

(2008). *Psicopatologia del senso comune.* Milan: Raffaello Cortina Editore.

(2009). Embodiment and schizophrenia. *World Psychiatry* 8: 56–59.

(2010). A hermeneutic framework for psychopathology. *Psychopathology* 43: 319–326.

(2011). Phenomenology: a method for care? *Philosophy, Psychiatry, & Psychology* 18: 25–29.

(2013a). The ethics of incomprehensibility. In G. Stanghellini and T. Fuchs (eds.), *One Century of Karl Jaspers' General Psychopathology*. Oxford University Press, pp. 166–183.

(2013b). Philosophical resources for the psychiatric interview. In K. W. M. Fulford, M. Davies, R. G. T. Gipps, G. Graham, J. Z. Sadler, G. Stanghellini, and T. Thornton (eds.), *The Oxford Handbook of Philosophy and Psychiatry*. Oxford University Press, pp. 321–356.

(2016a). *Lost in Dialogue: Anthropology, Psychopathology and Care*. Oxford University Press.

(2016b). Phenomenological psychopathology and care: from person-centered dialectical psychopathology to the PHD method for psychotherapy. In G. Stanghellini and M. Aragona (eds.), *An Experiential Approach to Psychopathology: What Is It Like to Suffer from Mental Disorders*. New York: Springer, pp. 361–378.

Stanghellini, G. and Ballerini, M. (2002). Dissociality: the phenomenological approach to social dysfunction in schizophrenia. *World Psychiatry* 1: 102–106.

(2004). Autism: disembodied existence. *Philosophy, Psychiatry, & Psychology* 11: 259–268.

(2007). Values in persons with schizophrenia. *Schizophrenia Bulletin* 33: 131–141.

(2008). Qualitative analysis: its use in psychopathological research. *Acta Psychiatrica Scandinavica* 117: 161–163.

(2011). What is it like to be a person with schizophrenia in the social world? A first-person perspective study on schizophrenic dissociality. Part 2. Methodological issues and empirical findings. *Psychopathology* 44: 183–192.

Stanghellini, G., Ballerini, M., Blasi, S., Mancini, M., Presenza, S., Raballo, A., and Cutting, J. (2014). The bodily self: a qualitative study of abnormal bodily phenomena in persons with schizophrenia. *Comprehensive Psychiatry* 55: 1703–1711.

Stanghellini, G., Ballerini, M., Fusar Poli, P., and Cutting, J. (2012). Abnormal bodily experiences may be a marker of early schizophrenia? *Current Pharmaceutical Design* 18: 392–398.

Stanghellini, G., Ballerini, M., and Lysaker, P. H. (2014). Autism rating scale. *Journal of Psychopathology* 20: 273–285.

Stanghellini, G., Ballerini, M., Presenza, S., Mancini, M., Northoff, G., and Cutting, J. (2016). Abnormal time experiences in major depression: an empirical qualitative study. *Psychopathology*. doi:10.1159/000452892.

Stanghellini, G., Ballerini, M., Presenza, S., Mancini, M., Raballo, A., Blasi, S., and Cutting, J. (2015). Psychopathology of lived time: abnormal time experience in persons with schizophrenia. *Schizophrenia Bulletin* 42: 45–55.

Stanghellini, G. and Bertelli, M. (2006). Assessing the social behaviour of unipolar depressives: the criteria for typus melancholicus. *Psychopathology* 39: 179–186.

Stanghellini, G., Bertelli, M., and Raballo, A. (2006). Typus melancholicus: personality structure and the characteristics of major unipolar depressive episode. *Journal of Affective Disorders* 93: 159–167.

Stanghellini, G., Bolton, D., and Fulford, W. K. (2013). Person-centered psychopathology of schizophrenia: building on Karl Jaspers' understanding of patient's attitude towards his illness. *Schizophrenia Bulletin* 39: 287–294.

Stanghellini, G., Castellini, G., Brogna, P., Faravelli, C., and Ricca, V. (2012). Identity and eating disorders (IDEA): a questionnaire evaluating identity and embodiment in eating disorder patients. *Psychopathology* 45: 147–158.

Stanghellini, G. and Lysaker, P. H. (2007). The psychotherapy of schizophrenia through the lens of phenomenology: intersubjectivity and the search for the recovery of first- and second-person awareness. *American Journal of Psychotherapy* 61: 163–179.

Stanghellini, G., Mancini, M., Castellini, G., and Ricca, V. (forthcoming). Eating disorders as disorders of embodiment and identity: theoretical and empirical perspectives. In H. McBride and J. Kwee (eds.), *Embodiment and Eating Disorders: A Handbook of Theory, Research, Prevention and Treatment*. London: Routledge.

Stanghellini, G. and Muscelli, C. (2007). Real persons' experience of contamination obsessions: hypotheses from a Strausian analysis. *South African Journal of Psychiatry* 13: 79–83.

Stanghellini, G. and Raballo, A. (2007). Exploring the margins of the bipolar spectrum: temperamental features of the typus melancholicus. *Journal of Affective Disorders* 100: 13–21.

(2015). Differential typology of delusions in major depression and schizophrenia: a critique to the unitary concept of "psychosis." *Journal of Affective Disorders* 171: 171–178.

Stanghellini, G. and Rosfort, R. (2013a). Borderline depression: a desperate vitality. *Journal of Consciousness Studies* 20: 153–177.

(2013b). *Emotions and Personhood: Exploring Fragility – Making Sense of Vulnerability*. Oxford University Press.

(2013c). Empathy as a sense of autonomy. *Psychopathology* 46: 337–344.

(2015). Disordered selves or persons with schizophrenia? *Current Opinion in Psychiatry* 28: 256–263.

Stanghellini, G. and Rossi, R. (2014). Pheno-phenotypes: a holistic approach to the psychopathology of schizophrenia. *Current Opinion in Psychiatry* 27: 236–241.

Stanghellini, G. and Rossi Monti, M. (2009a). Explication or explanation? *Philosophy, Psychiatry, & Psychology* 16: 237–239.

(2009b). *Psicologia del patologico: Una prospettiva fenomenologica-dinamica*. Milan: Raffaello Cortina Editore.

Stanghellini, G., Trisolini, F., Castellini, G., Ambrosini, A., Faravelli, C., and Ricca, V. (2014). Is feeling extraneous from one's own body a core vulnerability feature in eating disorders? *Psychopathology* 48: 18–24.

Stern, D. N. (1985/2000). *The Interpersonal World of the Infant: A View from Psychoanalysis and Developmental Psychology*. New York: Basic Books.

Stevens, A., Doidge, N., Goldbloom, D., Voore, P., and Farewell, J. (1999). Pilot study of televideo psychiatric assessment in an underserviced community. *American Journal of Psychiatry* 156: 783–785.

Stoudemire, A. (1998). *Clinical Psychiatry for Medical Students*. Philadelphia, PA: Lippincott Williams & Wilkins.

Straus, E. W. (1947). Disorders of personal time in depressive states. *Southern Medical Journal* 40: 254–259.

(1948). *On Obsession: A Clinical and Methodological Study* (Nervous and Mental Disease Monograph No. 73). Johnson Reprint.

(1958). Aesthesiology and hallucinations. In R. May, E. Angel, and H. Ellenberger (eds.), *Existence: A New Dimension in Psychiatry and Psychology*. New York: Basic Books, pp. 139–169.

Svenaeus, F. (2007). Do antidepressants affect the self? A phenomenological approach. *Medicine, Healthcare, and Philosophy* 10: 153–166.

Tan, J. O., Hope, T., Stewart, A., and Fitzpatrick, R. (2006a). Competence to make treatment decisions in anorexia nervosa: thinking processes and values. *Philosophy, Psychiatry, & Psychology* 13: 267–282.

(2006b). Studying penguins to understand birds. *Philosophy, Psychiatry, & Psychology* 13: 299–301.

Tasman, A., Kay J., and Lieberman, J. A. (1997). *Psychiatry*. Philadelphia, PA: Saunders.

Tatossian, A. (1975). Phénoménologie de la dépression. *Psychiatries* 21: 77–85.

(1979). Aspects phénoménologiques du temps humain en psychiatrie. Colloque de Vézelay, juin 1977. In Y. Pelicier (ed.), *La folie, le temps, la folie*. Paris: Union Générale d'édition, pp. 111–142.

(1983). Dépression, vécu dépressif et orientation thérapeutique. In Collectif (ed.), *La maladie depressive*. Paris: Ciba, pp. 277–293.

(1985). Phénoménologie et life-event. In J. Guyotat and P. Fedida (eds.), *Evénement et Psychopatologie*. Lyon/Paris: SIMEP.

Tavris, C. (1989). *Anger: The Misunderstood Emotion*, revised edition. New York: Simon & Schuster.

Tellenbach, H. (1961/1980). *Melancholy: History of the Problem, Endogeneity, Typology, Pathogenesis, Clinical Considerations*. Pittsburg, PA: Duquesne University Press.

(1968). *Geschmack und Atmosphäre*. Salzburg: Otto Müller Verlag.

Thompson, E. (2007). *Mind in Life*. Cambridge, MA: Harvard University Press.

Tozzi, F., Thornton, L. M., Klump, K. L., . . . and Kaye, W. H. (2005). Symptom fluctuation in eating disorders: correlates of diagnostic crossover. *American Journal of Psychiatry* 162: 732–740.

Troisi, A. (2011). Mental health and wellbeing: clinical applications of Darwinian psychiatry. In S. C. Roberts (ed.), *Applied Evolutionary Psychology*. Oxford University Press, pp. 276–289.

Troisi, A. and McGuire, M. (1998). *Darwinian Psychiatry*. Oxford University Press.

Turner, S. M. and Hersen, M. (2003). The interviewing process. In M. Hersen and S. M. Turner (eds.), *Diagnostic Interviewing*, 3rd edition. New York: Springer, pp. 3–11.

Urfer, A. (2001). Phenomenology and psychopathology of schizophrenia: the views of Eugène Minkowski. *Philosophy, Psychiatry, & Psychology* 8: 279–289.

van Praag, H. M., Asnis, G. M., Kahn, R. S., Brown, S. L., Korn, M., Friedman, J. M., and Wetzler, S. (1997). Nosological tunnel vision in biological psychiatry: a plea for functional psychopathology. *Annals of the New York Academy of Sciences* 600: 501–510.

Varela, F., Thompson, E., and Rosch, E. (1991). *The Embodied Mind*. Cambridge, MA: MIT Press.

Ventura, J., Liberman, R. P., Green, M. F., Shaner, A., and Mintz, J. (1998). Training and quality assurance with the Structured Clinical Interview for DSM-IV (SCID-I/P). *Psychiatric Research* 79: 163–173.

von Gebsattel, V. E. (1938). Die Welt des Zwangskranken. *Monatschrift für Psychiatrie und Neurologie* 99: 10–74.

(1954). *Prolegomena einer medizinischen Anthropologie*. Berlin: Springer.

von Weizsäcker, V. (1940). *Der Gestaltkreis*. Stuttgart: Thieme.

Ware, J., Straussman, H. D., and Naftulin, D. H. (1971). A negative relationship between understanding interviewing principles and interview performance. *Journal of Medical Education* 46: 620–622.

Westen, D. and Cohen, R. P. (1993). The self in borderline personality disorder: a psychodynamic perspective. In Z. V. Segal and S. J. Blatt (eds.), *The Self in Emotional Distress: Cognitive and Psychodynamic Perspectives*. New York: Guilford Press, pp. 334–368.

Westen, D., Novotny, C. M., and Thompson-Brenner, H. (2004). The empirical status of empirically supported psychotherapies: assumptions, findings, and reporting in controlled trials. *Psychological Bulletin* 130: 631–663.

Wilkinson-Ryan, T. and Westen, D. (2000). Identity disturbance in borderline personality disorder: an empirical investigation. *American Journal of Psychiatry* 157: 528–541.

Willi, J. (1999). *Ecological Developing by Shaping the Personal Niche*. Cambridge, MA: Hogrefe & Huber.

Williams, B. (1993). *Shame and Necessity*. Berkeley, CA: University of California Press.

Williams, G. J., Chamove, A. S., and Millar, H. R. (1990). Eating disorders, perceived control, assertiveness and hostility. *British Journal of Clinical Psychology* 29: 327–335.

Wittgenstein, L. (1953). *Philosophical Investigations*. New York: Macmillan.

Wolfe, B. E., Baker, C. W., Smith, A. T., and Kelly-Weeder, S. (2009). Validity and utility of the current definition of binge eating. *International Journal of Eating Disorders* 42: 674–686.

Woolgar, S. (1996). Psychology, qualitative methods and the ideas of science. In J. T. Richardson (ed.), *Handbook of Qualitative Research Methods for Psychology and the Social Sciences*. Leicester: British Psychological Society, pp. 11–24.

Yeats, W. B. (1991). *The Poems, Revised: The Collected Works of W. B . Yeats*. Berlin: Springer.

Yoshino, A., Shighemura, J., Kobayashi, Y., Nomura, S., Shishikura, K., . . . and Ashida, H. (2001). Telepsychiatry: assessment of televideo psychiatric interview reliability with present and next generation internet infrastructures. *Acta Psychiatrica Scandinavica* 104: 223–226.

Zahavi, D. (1999). *Self-Awareness and Alterity: A Phenomenological Investigation*. Evanston, IL: Northwestern University Press.

(2003). *Husserl's Phenomenology*. Stanford University Press.

(2005). *Subjectivity and Selfhood: Investigating the First-Person Perspective*. Cambridge, MA: MIT Press.

Zimmerman, M. (1993). A five-minute psychiatric screening interview. *Journal of the Family Practitioner* 37: 479–482.

Zinberg, N. E. (1987). Elements of the private therapeutic interview. *American Journal of Psychiatry* 144: 1527–1533.

Zutt, J. (1963). *Auf dem Wege zu einer anthropologischen Psychiatrie*. Berlin: Springer Verlag.

Index

Locators in **bold** refer to tables